"*Stronger than BPD* feels like a [...] while I learn practical tools tha[...] emotions."

—**Tamra Sattler, PhD, M** [...]
and entrepreneur

"Debbie has written a wise and wonderful book for those who struggle with borderline personality disorder (BPD). *Stronger than BPD* provides an honest look at recovery while inspiring all of us to be our very best through more skillful living. I'm exceptionally proud to recommend this book to my clients and their family members."

—**Amanda L. Smith, LMSW**, dialectical behavior therapist and treatment consultant, and author of *The Dialectical Behavior Therapy Wellness Planner*

"This book offers you a set of skills from someone who has been there. These are not theoretical experiences but instead the help and reflections that come from someone who has been there to those going through real-time struggles. A great addition to the literature."

—**Blaise Aguirre, MD**, medical director at McLean 3East Continuum of Care, assistant professor of psychiatry at Harvard Medical School, and coauthor of *Mindfulness for Borderline Personality Disorder*

"Written with the wisdom of one who has both suffered and lived in the solution, Debbie Corso's *Stronger than BPD* is a unique and highly accessible guide for those struggling with BPD traits, and the people who support them. Through powerful personal examples and with the clarity of a seasoned professional, Corso teaches the reader, step by step, to apply dialectical behavior therapy (DBT) skills to the storms of emotional turmoil and turbulent relationships. The author's hard-won success is an inspiration and testament to the power of DBT to heal and create lives truly worth living. Perfect as a stand-alone workbook as well as a complement to clinical support, *Stronger than BPD* is a remarkable guide that will change lives and bring new understanding to the practice of DBT."

—**Kiera Van Gelder, MFA**, author of the highly
acclaimed memoir, *The Buddha and the Borderline*

"DBT is touted by thousands of clinicians all over the globe. This book raises the bar because it describes survivors' lived experience—the most important testimonial of all. Congratulations to Debbie!"

—**Perry D. Hoffman, PhD**, president and cofounder
of the National Education Alliance for Borderline
Personality Disorder (NEA.BPD)

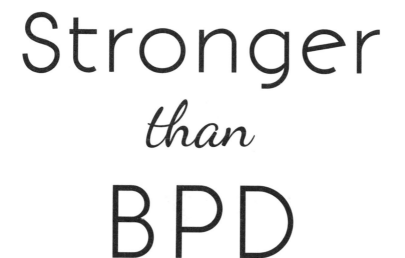

Stronger
than
BPD

THE *Girl's Guide* TO
**TAKING CONTROL OF INTENSE EMOTIONS,
DRAMA & CHAOS USING DBT**

DEBBIE CORSO

New Harbinger Publications, Inc.

Publisher's Note

Distributed in Canada by Raincoast Books

Copyright © 2017 by Debbie Corso
New Harbinger Publications, Inc.
5674 Shattuck Avenue
Oakland, CA 94609
www.newharbinger.com

Cover design by Amy Shoup

Acquired by Jess O'Brien

Edited by Brady Kahn

All Rights Reserved

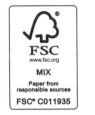

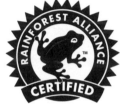

Library of Congress Cataloging-in-Publication Data on file

19   18   17

10   9   8   7   6   5   4   3   2   1   First Printing

Contents

Foreword   v

Introduction   1

chapter 1   Paying Attention to Your Life (on Purpose)   15

chapter 2   Coping Effectively with Distress   59

chapter 3   Regulating Your Emotions   83

chapter 4   Working on Relationships   117

chapter 5   Putting It All Together   165

Thank You   169

References   173

Foreword

The practice of dialectical behavioral therapy (DBT) can seem deceptively simple. Many non-DBT therapists will talk about DBT as just a set of skills that you need to learn. In fact, this is how you may have been sold on DBT.

However, when you choose to embark on the journey of DBT, you quickly find that learning the skills is the easy part. Most people find learning the DBT skills relatively straightforward: some skills are more intuitive than others and some perhaps a bit more confusing; some people get lost in the multitude of acronyms, while others find the acronyms the easiest way to keep the many skills in mind.

The challenge comes after you learn the skills—when you have to use them in your life and in our fast-paced culture, with its high levels of stimulation and instant gratification. You'll find you have little time to consult your skills manual when responding to a text message or setting a limit or an expectation with your boss. The immediacy of daily life means it's hard to respond without losing your cool or, worse, losing your self-respect. Skill takes time to build. What we know is that the best way to begin to be skillful is to practice—practice new, more effective ways to live your life and manage your emotions. Practice means that you must risk messing up, getting it wrong, or—maybe the scariest possibility—letting your emotions get the best of you one more time.

As you persist in practicing DBT, you will not become a new person. Rather, you will gain the skills you need to manage the parts of your life that currently feel unmanageable. The more you practice doing things ineffectively, the better you get at being ineffective. Fortunately, the more you practice being effective, the more effective you become. This link between practice and skill is one of the few simple things about our very complicated brains, and it is good news. Even older brains can change and rewire.

This book is a wonderful companion if you are in a DBT therapy. I have had the pleasure of working with Debbie as she has written this book. Her own experiences, and her passion and dedication to healing through the use of DBT, shine through each page. Debbie humbly shares her own experience as she teaches you the intricacies of both learning DBT, and, more importantly, applying it to your life. This book offers you a set of skills, real-life examples of when they work, and the roadblocks that you may run into. A little humor takes the edge off some of Debbie's own challenging, and sometimes painful, learning experiences. As you embark on this path of skill-building and healing, Debbie stands alongside you.

It is quite a gift not only to be taught DBT by a professional, but also to augment your journey with the company and support of someone who has been there. I often tell my clients that sometimes it takes a village to support you making these changes, so look for people and resources in your life that will support you.

Wishing you a skillful and mindful journey.

—Gillian Galen, PsyD
  Program Director
  3East Adolescent Intensive Residential Program
  McLean Hospital
  Instructor in Psychology
  Harvard Medical School Department of Psychiatry

Introduction

What's more upsetting than being told you're a drama queen (or king)—or that you always need to be the center of attention and that you thrive on chaos and crisis—possibly because at least a tiny bit of you knows that there is truth in the accusation? That was the question on the table for me yet again. My boss couldn't understand my emotional reaction—or "breakdown," as I believe he called it—in response to an escalation of stressful deadlines at work. A few days prior, we were out in the field visiting customers and vendors, and I hadn't eaten enough, which caused a scary episode of low blood sugar. I felt weak and dizzy and had tremors all over. It was preventable, but self-care was not something I typically thought about at that time of my life. I had been anxious and didn't feel like eating, so I didn't. I didn't plan ahead or think of how I would deal with the consequences of that choice or that there might, in fact, be any.

And, just as I had not been making my physical health a priority, I wasn't doing so well with my mental health either, and this evidently was experienced by the outside world as my being dramatic—at least, that was the feedback I was receiving. A few days later, lying on a hospital cot with an oxygen sensor on my right index finger and an IV tube with saline fluids going into my left arm, I didn't really have a whole lot of insight into how I had ended up once again in the emergency room. I would find myself at the ER all too often, as my emotional state would get to the point where it felt like a life-or-death situation, a real emergency. I was in the ER that time because I had become dehydrated after being in a state of mental crisis, but I didn't understand any of this then.

I didn't know why I responded to stress and anxiety the way I did, and I didn't have the conscious awareness to consider the effects or impact of my behavior on my life and on others. That is, I didn't have the awareness that I have now, in retrospect. In fact, all I could think of at that time of my life, in that moment on the cot and in general, was that I needed someone to save me, and fast. From my past. From my present. From myself. And, in all fairness, maybe I was a little dramatic. What's more dramatic than being a regular at the emergency room, right?

If you have also been accused of being a drama queen or king, please go easy on yourself. You're not being that way without reason—there is an explanation—and you probably just don't know how to rein in your intense emotions yet.

What I learned, and what you may very well relate to from your own experience, is this: I felt desperate. Desperate for someone to convince me that I was and would be okay. That I was safe. Desperate for someone to comfort and reassure me that I would make it through my episodes of emotional pain. That I wasn't in this thing called "life" all alone. My twin fears of rejection and abandonment formed the driving force behind all my choices, but no one had drawn this connection yet, including myself. And my desperation played itself out in some dramatic ways, like ending up in the ER over and over again. Your dramatic scene may play out differently, but it's that core driving force that so many of us with borderline personality disorder, BPD traits, or emotional sensitivity have in common. We're afraid of being rejected and abandoned, and we want someone else to rescue us. We don't trust or have faith in our own power to rescue ourselves. This was my story.

On the day of this particular ER visit—and for many years of my life—I didn't feel safe unless I was in a clinical environment surrounded by gods and goddesses (also known as doctors and nurses) who could care for me and watch over me. I revered my clinical team in this way and also thought of them as my posse. My friends. My family. And, in fact, for many years, they were my main support system. I simply had no confidence in my ability to get myself through an emotional crisis on my own or that it might even be possible to do so. My version of self-care was to look outside of myself for someone else to make everything okay. I was dependent and needy, and although deep down I knew this to be true and I felt helpless and hopeless to ever change, the very words "dependent" and "needy"—or, God forbid, being accused of being them—caused me to cringe and lash out. If this sounds all too familiar, please have compassion for yourself, right where you are, in this moment of your ever-evolving journey. We get caught up in learned patterns. We get stuck sometimes. We need to learn new ways to better take care of ourselves. Sometimes, despite how strong we are, we still need help. I have been no exception.

And there I was again, dehydrated after becoming so worked up emotionally that I couldn't keep anything down. My nervous system had once again gone into red alert. You've been there, right? Getting yourself so anxious and worked up that you end up feeling physically sick as well, which only serves to drive the anxiety more and more and cause you to feel inconsolable? That's where I was. I was, for the umpteenth time, unknowingly reliving trauma from my past, incidents that likely helped greatly in setting the stage for my developing borderline personality disorder: trauma involving feeling more alone than any human being, let alone a child, should ever feel. Utterly abandoned. Terrified. Each time that memories or flashbacks from the past trauma would arise in the here and now, as an adult, I would become emotionally dysregulated beyond comprehension. For many years, I also did not have the insight to make the connection between the trauma drama I was experiencing as an adult and the triggering, long ingrained trauma of the past.

You may be nodding your head up and down right about now, having been there yourself many times. If you have borderline personality disorder, BPD traits, or are emotionally sensitive, you may also have, as I do, complex post-traumatic stress syndrome (CPTSD), which causes episodes that, without skills to manage them effectively, can feel as if we are reliving the trauma of the past, all over again, in the here and now. It's very exhausting and difficult to bear, to say the least, both for us as the sufferers and for those who love and care about us. Loved ones may have a difficult time understanding why you're so upset during such an episode. You may hear the words, "Nothing bad is happening right now" or "That stuff happened over twenty years ago. Get over it!" An invalidating comment like either of these can send you spiraling further into fear and despair, right? That place of helplessness where you just desperately want someone to truly understand the heaviness of your anguish and to comfort you, not dismiss your experience as a cry for attention or a display of melodrama. And people mean well. Our loved ones tend to want to make things better, to get us to snap out of the negative mental space we're in, so we don't cause more damage to ourselves. If only it were that easy.

Back in the emergency room, I had well-meaning loved ones around, too. But when it came to my experience of the severe mental dysregulation that comes with being in the thick of BPD and CPTSD symptomatology, this just wasn't enough. I needed an intervention of a clinical caliber. I ended up in this crisis situation, yet again, because I did not know how to regulate my emotions. This lack of control led to my acting out in ways that I would often regret, further perpetuating the dysregulated state. Namely, I engaged in self-defeating behaviors that ended up pushing others away, creating circumstances that were the direct opposite of what I longed for, and feeding into the deep fears I held about rejection and abandonment from past wounds. These self-sabotaging acts also made it difficult to stick with school, a job, or meaningful relationships with others, for any length of time. I would seem to do well for short periods, only to find myself back in crisis survival "rescue me" mode again and again, essentially fitting the description of an unstable person.

The truth is, we can only work with the tools and knowledge that we have. We do what seems to work until it doesn't anymore, and that's where I was. At this point, though, I was finally motivated enough to break the cycle. Fortunately, life was ready to meet me where I was, and this emergency room visit ultimately led to me being referred to something called dialectical behavior therapy (DBT). It was only a few years ago that, with this newly gained knowledge of DBT skills under my belt, I dealt head-on with any of my past trauma.

As I mentioned, my insights into my experiences of emotion, behavior, and consequences up until then had ranged from nonexistent to severely limited. Knowing what I now know, I realize that it is a deep understanding and consistent daily practice of DBT skills that has made dealing with past trauma even possible. I had tried a trauma recovery group before learning these skills and was unable to stick with it. The range and intensity of my emotions was too much to bear, and I could not adequately cope or comfort myself. I needed to learn how to not be destroyed by emotional pain and suffering in the here and now before I could visit my past with bravery and find some healing and closure there. Enter DBT.

Dialectical Behavior Therapy

Dialectical behavior therapy is a set of often very highly effective skills, developed originally by Marsha Linehan (1993a, 1993b, 2014a, 2014b) to treat chronic suicidality in patients diagnosed with borderline personality disorder by helping them learn to manage their emotions; it is now being used more widely to help many people who identify as being emotionally sensitive or otherwise emotionally dysregulated. Before I had access to these godsend skills, I tried not to think about my past trauma. I suppressed it. But, as all of us who have trauma in our past eventually find out, trying to squelch, squash, deny, or silence a traumatic incident doesn't make it go away. It doesn't undo it. It doesn't help us cope effectively.

In fact, in a desperate attempt to be heard and healed, the trauma will continuously manage to show up in different ways, including sometimes through threats of suicide and repeated self-sabotage. This is another common trait of those with BPD: frequent threats of suicide, sometimes acting on those threats, and engaging in acts of self-harm, whether physical or through self-sabotage. There were times when I thought I wanted to die because of the emotional pain I was experiencing, but after recovering from episodes of severe dysregulation, I realized that saying I wanted to die and feeling suicidal, for me, wasn't truly about wanting life to end. It was about wanting the pain to end, and my threats were a plea for help. When I felt well, I loved life. I would hold on to this truth in the moments of my deepest despair and then seek help. Going to the emergency room was a cry for help, rooted in deep, unhealed, trauma-related pain.

Though I personally chose to apply my newly learned skills in a trauma recovery group, practicing DBT isn't necessarily about going back and healing old wounds. It's actually more about coping in an effective way now and moving forward in ways that allow you to lead the life you want to lead as an emotionally sensitive person. And, whether you have past trauma to deal with or not, you most likely have plenty of stuff to sort out, deal with, and heal from in the present. That's where these skills can be critically helpful. Until we have them in our toolbox, we can feel utterly ill-equipped for coping with unpredictable life in the here and now.

Before finding DBT, I guess you could say that I had hit my emotional rock bottom. I had sabotaged yet another job, and the only two people I hadn't completely alienated in my life were giving me a tough-love ultimatum: "Stop doing this to yourself, or I can't be there for you anymore." This threat both terrified me and served as a wake-up call. I needed to gain control of my life. I needed to change the way that I handled (or rather, didn't handle) my life when stress—something that seemed completely unmanageable to me, even in small doses—came up. The alternative scenario, namely losing the last two people in my life and ending up eternally unemployed or hopping from job to job, was simply unbearable and unacceptable. I needed help, and it was no longer something I could deny.

But how? How would I ever break free of the constant drama, chaos, and crisis that I knew as life? If, in my early thirties, I hadn't yet figured out a different way to be, what miracle was going to show up and change the course of my life? These questions had just been going through my head when the on-call psychiatrist showed up at my ER bedside and told me that he thought I needed to go into an intensive outpatient program. This is essentially a psychiatric hospital experience during the day, where you get to go home in the evening and on the weekends. He didn't feel I needed inpatient treatment, but he definitely knew I needed something intensive. I agreed.

That evening I decided that I could no longer go on the way I'd been going. I didn't know how I was going to change the course of my life. I just knew that I had to. In this outpatient program, I would lay all my cards on the table: my thoughts (as distorted and insane as some of them felt and might have sounded to someone else), my experience of being terrified at the thought of being alone, even for short amounts of time, and, perhaps most troubling, the fact that I didn't have a clear sense of self but described myself as a "shape-shifting chameleon." I would later learn that this is known as *identity disturbance* and is one of the possible criteria for borderline personality disorder.

In my case, it was as if I were a teenager who never outgrew the stage of trying to find her identity by experimenting with different peer groups. I was so suggestible and chameleon-like that I would align with my gung ho Republican friends in one conversation, only to be completely converted in a matter of hours to a die-hard left-wing liberal. I became like others around me, matching up to their mannerisms and becoming who I thought they wanted me to be, all in an effort to be liked, accepted, and to not be rejected. Music styles, recreational activities, religious beliefs, sexual orientation preferences—nothing was off-limits for my constantly shifting sense of self.

It was frightening to imagine being in the same room with all of the people I knew. I wouldn't know who to be or how to behave, since each of them knew me to be someone who was just like them. I wasn't sure that I could ever overcome this particular aspect of BPD, but I did. Through dedicated learning and a consistent, diligent practice of DBT skills, it has been possible for me and many others I know to overcome issues like this one that initially seemed insurmountable.

So, you might be wondering if DBT managed to fix everything in my life and if it is going to be the solution that wholly fixes yours. The answer is no, and quite frankly, I'm not so sure that all of what we struggle with and think we need to change actually needs fixing. In many ways, I've learned to embrace the difficult parts of my personality and appreciate the benefits of having gone from a person who was completely out of control and at the mercy of her emotions to someone who remains emotionally sensitive, who still experiences her feelings intensely but who now has tools to skillfully handle them so that she no longer needs to be marked as fragile—by myself, professionals, peers, and loved ones. I was always and continue to be an emotionally sensitive person. Without skills to manage the intensity that can come with this way of being, I found myself in chaos. Feelings were so strong that I was overcome by them. I would routinely feel emotionally dysregulated and unable to manage ordinary, let alone moderate to severe, distress. Today I can feel my emotions and not be derailed or destroyed by them. The goal is not to not feel. It's to feel, function, and thrive.

During my time in the intensive outpatient program, I learned that I did, in fact, have borderline personality disorder. I finally had an accurate diagnosis, which led to learning that there was a treatment (DBT) designed specifically to help those with this disorder and that I could have access to it. I committed to dialectical behavior therapy like nothing before in my life. I wanted it to work. I needed it to work. It had worked for others, so I was convinced that if I committed to the program, completely subscribed to the teachings, and applied what I learned to my life, it would work for me. It had to. It was my last hope. The good news is, it did.

DBT changed and saved my life. I devoted myself to learning the skills and applying them, and my passion is to share my journey with others who are looking to make a monumental shift of breaking free of drama, chaos, and crisis and embracing life as emotionally sensitive people. I teach as a peer educator at DBT Path, an entirely online, DBT-informed psychoeducational school that I founded and which has global attendance. Each week, I cofacilitate classes with a licensed therapist and encourage other emotionally sensitive people to change their lives and overcome so much more than they may have previously imagined possible.

You are about to dig into a book that could truly change your life. In it, I'll describe how DBT skills can be applied in many of the common situations that we face as people who easily become emotionally dysregulated. I primarily give personal examples, but I also draw upon stories I've heard while teaching at DBT Path as well as while interacting with my blog readers. You may relate to many of these stories on a deep level. My hope is that you will feel inspired and hopeful about taking charge of your life, leaving a victim mentality behind, and setting out on your own personal path of healing.

In the chapters that follow, we'll be digging into four main DBT skill sets: paying attention to your life (on purpose); coping effectively with distress (going from "I can't handle this" to "I am handling this"); regulating your emotions; and working on important relationships. All of these skills, drawn from Marsha Linehan's work (1993a, 1993b, 2014a, 2014b), can help you deal with the things that would otherwise dysregulate you. We are going to dig deep! Because I am a peer educator and not a psychologist or doctor, this book is not meant as a substitute for psychiatric or medical care, but it can serve as an inspirational part of your journey. If you are seeing a therapist, you can discuss how the various exercises that you complete can be used as opportunities to learn, grow, and change your life.

BPD and Emotional Sensitivity

Throughout this book, I'll be referring to both borderline personality disorder and emotional sensitivity. I have a history of being diagnosed with BPD, and I continue to meet some of the diagnostic criteria but not enough for a diagnosis and am therefore said to be in recovery or in remission. However, because I had borderline personality disorder for likely over a decade before receiving my official diagnosis, and I continue to live with BPD traits, I can genuinely relate to where you are if you struggle with this disorder. I hope this book reassures you that you are not alone and that there is real hope for you, too.

Additionally, I have always considered myself to be an emotionally sensitive person. I don't believe this will ever change, nor do I want it to. I experience my emotions intensely and experience empathy on a deep level, and both, when channeled skillfully, have led to creative endeavors and projects that have allowed for cathartic self-expression and have helped others. I embrace my emotional sensitivity and will be encouraging you to do the same. Emotional sensitivity and emotional dysregulation are not exclusive to BPD but can be part of many psychological diagnoses. They can also be present in people in the absence of any diagnosis. So you do not need to have a BPD diagnosis to learn and potentially experience immense benefits from practicing dialectical behavior therapy skills. Many of my students come from different backgrounds, including having bipolar disorder, identifying as highly sensitive, or having intense emotional sensitivity or emotion dysregulation patterns but without any formal diagnosis.

So, go out and get yourself a nice new notebook and pen and create some time and space dedicated to your own well-being and self-discovery. There will be exercises for you to practice and journal. Let's get started!

Chapter 1

Paying Attention to Your Life (on Purpose)

It's time to get started learning some of the DBT skills that have helped countless others like us reclaim their sanity, reduce self-sabotaging, and find more emotional balance and contentment. We'll start at the very beginning, at the foundation of all of the skills, with something called mindfulness. A fundamental understanding and practice of mindfulness skills will be at the core of successfully practicing each and every DBT skill you learn. This is not a topic to simply be skimmed. As Blaise Aguirre, MD, and Gillian Galen, PsyD, point out in their helpful text on this subject, "Many people with BPD have found mindfulness to be the way out of their suffering" (Aguirre and Galen 2013, 29). This chapter will be the longest and most comprehensive one in this book. You'll be returning to the concepts presented here, time and time again, as a resource to help you practice the skills in ways proven to yield the most benefit.

The Power of Mindfulness

So what does mindfulness mean in the context of DBT? The term *mindfulness* is quite overused in our society, sometimes causing the concept to feel somewhat clichéd. New Age music, some candles, and a drumming circle, anyone? Actually, that sounds like fun, but I digress. It's important that, as emotionally sensitive people, we not dismiss the significant impact that a mindfulness practice can have on our lives and emotional well-being. Many people with BPD or emotional sensitivity find behaving mindfully to be a meaningful and powerful catalyst into a mental space that allows for self-reflection, connection with one's true self, and a source of emotional balance and peace. Through the mindfulness skills of awareness, attention, and conscious redirection of the mind, DBT teaches us to focus all of our attention on one thing at a time while remaining aware of the greater context of what is happening in that moment. That's it. Nothing super complicated. Nothing ultramystical. But it does take practice and conscious effort, and not all moments will be as easy as others to mindfully live in.

Add to this that we live in a world where doing one thing at a time is rarely encouraged. We need to actively and consistently work to develop this ability. The reward of such hard work is worth it. Don't worry—you'll still be able to multitask in those situations where there is no getting around it, but as you bring more and more mindfulness to other areas of your life, you will likely notice a major difference between the quality of your attention and the outcomes of the activities in which you multitask and the quality of your attention and the outcomes of those that you do one at a time. If anything, this will probably encourage you to bring mindful attention to one thing at a time as much as you possibly can.

Beyond noticing a higher quality of attention and better results in what we do, being mindful through our conscious, deliberate focusing of attention allows us, as emotionally sensitive people, to experience something very practical that will help us thrive in this world: we learn how to *respond* rather than *react*. This reduces our emotional suffering and potentially improves the important relationships in our lives, which is something that you'll probably agree is a huge motivating factor for learning these skills in the first place. In the meantime, as we work up to this ability, we get to practice on a daily basis to really build up our mindfulness muscle.

As I began to apply conscious redirection of my attention on routine activities that were once mundane, and which I robotically or mysteriously achieved during the day (for example, driving home from the grocery store or washing and conditioning my hair in the shower), suddenly those activities became magical and more meaningful. I began noticing what was coming through my five senses in each daily activity and realized how much I was missing by living my life on autopilot or by constantly getting deeply caught up in and distracted by the past and the future worry stories in my mind. At first, I honestly didn't understand how something like mindfully driving, taking a shower, or eating a piece of fruit would have an impact on my emotional dysregulation and suffering and how it could possibly help. You might be wondering that, too. I even balked at this set of teachings, but since I was in a place of desperation and needed DBT to work for me, I reminded myself of my commitment to truly adhere to the lessons I was being taught, trusting that if the skills worked for others before me, I could expect to see benefits if I applied myself.

As it turned out, thankfully, my efforts were not in vain, and I expect yours will not be either. In fact, the payoffs have been so nice and worthwhile that I feel fueled and motivated to continue living my life in a mindful manner. This is not to say that I am *always* mindful, and please do not hold that unrealistic expectation for yourself, either. For the most part, however, I now have a really good awareness of when I stray from being mindful into mindlessness, and then in that paradoxical moment, I become mindful again. With patience and a willingness to keep practicing the mindfulness skills that you are about to learn, I saw the benefits continue to unfold and become obvious, as I believe they will for you, too.

One of the biggest benefits is that as we learn about mindfulness, grasp the concepts of it, and begin applying its principles to our lives on a daily basis, we empower ourselves to be equipped to best handle whatever may present itself to us in the moment, including an intense emotion, troubling or triggering situation, upsetting thought, memory from the past, or worry about the future. An important aspect of being mindful means being aware of what we are experiencing in *this* moment. We may have a *thought* about something tragic that happened to us in the past, but mindfulness allows us to remember that we are not experiencing that tragedy right now. In this moment, we are safe.

In this moment, we are grown and able to take care of ourselves and to keep ourselves out of harm's way. In this moment, we are only having a thought about the past—we are not experiencing the issue again and are not *in* the past. This is a huge distinction that can take time to develop but ultimately leads to substantially reducing our suffering. When I began to remind myself of this truth while experiencing memories of childhood abuse, it would help me to not go as deep into dissociation and despair as I had in the past. Without mindfulness, my mind would continue to spiral deeper into the pain and terror of those moments as if I were reliving them all over again, as is typical in complex post-traumatic stress disorder. With mindfulness of this moment, I can now separate my present experience from the thought and its accompanying intense emotions. I don't have to suffer the past over and over. I didn't know this before, which led to an incredible amount of my time being lived in emotional dysregulation and despair.

What I've learned through practicing mindfulness is that if we pay attention to this moment and all that is happening in it, we become aware that several things are often competing for our attention, including our physical sensations, emotions and feelings, and thoughts. Sometimes our thoughts are about things that are happening in this moment, but more often than not, our brains like to time travel to a past that continues to trouble us (such as my ruminations on past trauma) or to an unknown future that worries us (the famous *what ifs?*).

Past and future thoughts inevitably rob us of joy, and they take us out of the experience we are having right now. Part of mindfulness is noticing when our thoughts take us to the past or the future. This is a practice that most people on this planet aren't exploring. It is hard work, and you may notice that as you begin to practice and see changes in your life, others will wonder what you are doing differently, and you may begin to have an increased sense of compassion for those who are continuing to live their lives in an unconsciously mindless manner. Everyone is on his or her unique journey, and as Maya Angelou once put it so aptly, "Do the best you can until you know better. Then when you know better, do better." That's all we can expect from others or ourselves, right?

With this newfound ability to bring awareness of where our minds are at any given time and an awareness and nonjudgmental acceptance that not everyone else is actively working on these skills alongside us, we can then take the next step. We can choose to notice where our mind has gone, acknowledge the drifting, and then bring ourselves back to experiencing what is happening in this very moment—and this includes the difficult moments. These can be more of a challenge, and we often need to develop advanced mindfulness skills to grasp why we would even want to acknowledge, accept, and work through a painful moment rather than simply push it away and avoid the pain. This book will help you get to this point as you learn a variety of mindfulness techniques. It all begins with acknowledging that pain and suffering are very different. There is truth in the old saying that pain is inevitable but suffering is optional. And pushing painful experiences away only gives them strength. This will make more sense the more you learn and practice mindfulness.

Taking the First Step

Mindfulness is an invaluable tool to help us break free from patterns of chaos and drama. But before you pick up this tool and learn to use it, you may need to dispel any myths you have about what mindfulness is. Prior to reading this book, when you heard the word "mindfulness," what images came to mind? Prior to DBT, when I heard the word, I pictured so many things. I thought that to practice I'd need some type of altar with lit candles and chanting music in the background. I thought that I might need to consider converting or subscribing to some type of spiritual path or religious teaching. While some who practice mindfulness may find any or all of the things I pictured to be helpful on their own personal paths, DBT presents mindfulness in a secular way that allows for anyone to practice without infringing on your personal spiritual or religious preferences.

So if you've been afraid to practice mindfulness because you've been concerned that it is contrary to your religion or that it is "out there," I have two pieces of good news: it isn't, and nearly all of the world's religious and spiritual practices actually encourage mindful living. Now with that potential objection or concern set aside, let's take a look at what mindfulness looks like in the context of practicing as part of dialectical behavior therapy. In just a moment, I will ask you to place this book or electronic reading device down on the table. We are going to jump right in with a quick, simple activity.

Real-World Activity:
Basic Mindfulness Practice

Read the instructions, and then place your book down to practice the task. When you've completed the task, resume reading.

Instructions: It's time to pull out your notebook and pen to record your experience during your first formal mindfulness practice. Set a timer for two minutes, so you can focus on the practice while not worrying about keeping track of time. With your eyes open with a soft gentle gaze, look at the floor about two to three feet ahead of you or at a boring spot on the wall. Now, bring your attention to your breath. Place one hand on your chest and the other on your abdomen, just below your sternum. Notice which part rises and which part falls as you inhale and exhale. Do this until the timer goes off, and then return to your reading.

So what did you notice? Jot down what you noticed in your notebook. You may note any of the following:

- your breath
- distracting thoughts
- sounds in your environment
- feeling bored
- feeling tired
- something else

Great job. You just completed the first mindfulness practice of this book. Are you doubting that you completed it correctly? Here's the great thing about mindfulness practice: if you noticed anything about your experience, it was a success! Sure, there is often a goal or an objective with a particular practice, in this case to pay attention to your breath, but if during this time you noticed distracting thoughts arise, sounds in your environment, feeling bored, feeling tired, or something else, you were mindfully aware of your experience. You did it. The underlying goal is to practice bringing your attention back to the task at hand whenever you notice that your mind has wandered to something else, which it inevitably, repeatedly will.

How Mindful Living Helps

So, why is mindful living so important for those of us who experience intense emotions? Mindful living allows us to insert a pause between having an intense thought or feeling and taking any action. This mindful pause can prevent us from engaging in the kind of knee-jerk reaction that has caused us so much pain and regret up until now. Part of the problem with emotional intensity that is not regulated through skillful intervention is that we often resort to unskillful, unhealthy, impulsive behaviors that defeat our goals and cause us more unnecessary emotional pain. The empowerment that you will experience when you begin to notice that you are making skillful, mindful choices is something that can't adequately be put into words. It's quite amazing and reinforces our desire to choose skillfully the next time, too. And, this is how a new habit—a new, mindful way of living—is born.

Again, it is important to acknowledge to yourself that you have been doing the best that you can with what you have known up until now. Please have compassion for yourself as you learn these skills and begin practicing them in your life. There will be times when an urge or impulse will be really strong and will test your dedication to practicing mindfulness techniques. When this happens, do your best to insert that skillful pause and allow yourself the opportunity to make a different choice. The more success you have in practicing skillfulness over unskillfulness, the greater your confidence and ability will be to build the life you want to live. And it will take practice! To put it in perspective, monks in Tibet are *still* practicing. And they dedicate their lives, 24/7, to mindfulness practice.

There is actually no shortage of opportunities to practice mindfulness. Formal sitting practices, like the one you did a few moments ago, focusing on the breath, are intended to prepare you to apply this type of focused attention to activities that you perform throughout the day. They are training exercises for bringing the quality of mindfulness to each and every moment of your life.

Real-World Activity:
Informal Mindfulness Practice

Choose an ordinary, everyday activity that you will perform in the next twenty-four hours. For example, it could be washing the dishes, making your bed, preparing dinner, or playing with your children. Pick your activity, and jot it down in your notebook.

Set the intention that you will focus your complete attention on the task at hand. If you choose to wash the dishes, just wash the dishes. No ruminating over thoughts or trying to solve problems in your head. No turning on music or talk radio. Just wash the dishes. Decide that you will focus your undivided attention on being completely and totally present with what is happening in that moment with that task. When you notice distracting thoughts arise, just notice them and then allow them to be released. You might picture yourself placing each thought on a leaf and allowing it to flow down the river or placing each thought on a cloud and watching it drift away. Do the same for any other distractions that arise within, and then mindfully, deliberately return your focus to the task at hand. It doesn't matter if you need to repeat this process a hundred times in the course of ten minutes. Just be sure to notice your experience with as little self-judgment as possible.

Once you've completed the activity, record what happened in your notebook and consider other everyday activities that you can practice mindfully, like this:

Activity: Washed the Dishes Mindfully

Time spent: *About ten minutes*

Things I noticed:

- *Mindful participation in my activity*
- *Distracting thoughts*
- *Sounds in my environment*
- *Feeling bored*
- *Feeling tired*

The next activity to which I will bring mindful attention is making the bed.

And I will practice this tomorrow morning.

Using this format, you can log your progress as you stick with mindful tasks longer and with greater ease.

———————————

You might be wondering why you would even want to bother practicing being mindful while doing ordinary, routine things throughout your day. After all, you could play with the kids while surfing social media on your phone and while texting your best friend. The thing is, you'd be missing out on those moments that will inevitably end up mattering the most. You will notice things about your children, their mannerisms, their facial expressions and body language, their preferences and personalities, so much more if you devote those moments fully to being present with them. So while practicing mindfulness while washing the dishes, driving, or making the bed may seem to have little value, these are actually great opportunities for turning your mind to focus on where you want it to be, so you will be more effective in doing so in situations that mean more to you.

Applying Mindfulness in the Real World

Now that you've done a couple of mindfulness practices, I'd like to share an example of a real-world application of this skill in my own life. Once in a great while, I have insomnia. If you've ever had difficulty getting enough sleep to feel rested and restored, you can probably remember the feeling of helplessness as you kept looking over at the clock, counting the hours until the alarm would go off and you'd have to get up for work, school, or other activities and responsibilities. You can probably remember the irritability you experienced throughout the sleepless night and into the following day and how your tolerance for any type of frustration was greatly diminished. These are not easy feelings to endure. We need sleep!

Often on sleepless nights, my automatic, learned, unskillful response was to resist the insomnia. You can imagine how that went! I would toss and turn and mumble angrily about how unfair it was that I was up at 3:00 a.m. I would lie awake in bed and hope that I would fall back to sleep. Sometimes I'd turn on my iPad and scroll through Facebook and other social media sites for hours. This did not help. I was left feeling frustrated, anxious, and already worrying about whether I'd make it through the day without collapsing. All of this was very unmindful and ultimately unproductive for getting some much-needed rest.

Let me be clear that bringing mindfulness to this particular situation did help but it didn't always result in getting the hours of lost sleep that I so desperately coveted. It did, however, result in *less emotional suffering*, which made it worth the effort. A conscious choice to deliberately apply mindfulness to the issue of insomnia and accept the possibility of not being able to sleep looked like this. At 10:30 p.m., I would shut off all electronic devices, thirty minutes ahead of when I would lie down. As someone who loves to be online, this was one of the most difficult things for me to do, but I knew from various health sources that this step is part of good sleep habits, such as avoiding caffeine at least six hours before you plan to go to bed and avoiding bright lights like those from electronic screens (McKay, Wood, and Brantley 2007). Some even suggest starting this ritual an hour before bed, but I haven't been ready to embrace that quite yet. The only exception was I used my iPad, with the screen covered and closed, to play a progressive muscle relaxation practice or a guided meditation while (hopefully) drifting off. And I'd inevitably drift.

Fast-forward several hours, and I would awaken, feeling confused that it was only 2:00 a.m. Why was I wide awake? With mindfulness, I would notice the anxiety rising up within me. I would pay attention to the feeling of my shoulders, jaw, and neck tightening and aching slightly. I would notice my thoughts: *Here we go again. It's only 2:00 a.m. What if I don't get enough sleep tonight? I have a meeting in the morning. How am I going to function?* Instead of getting caught up in each of those thoughts and engaging with them, I would practice an exercise I learned in DBT. I imagined myself floating above a conveyor belt, watching each of my thoughts, feelings, and physical sensations (whatever I noticed) coming down the conveyer belt below me. Whatever I noticed coming down the conveyor belt, I would sort by category into the appropriately labeled bucket: worry thoughts, thoughts about work, thoughts about my health, thoughts about relationships, appointment thoughts, deadline thoughts, and so on. As a thought came in, it got sorted. Thought: *What if I don't get enough sleep tonight?* Into the worry thought bucket you go.

The image of the conveyer belt helped me release these unproductive thoughts and sensations. It's so tempting to try to answer your 2:00 a.m. questions in a logical way, hoping that if you'll just satisfy your anxious mind's anxiety, it will bid you goodnight and you'll drift off into restful sleep, but this isn't usually what happens. If anything, when I engaged my thoughts in the middle of the night, I found that while I may have started out coming up with a rational, logical answer to myself, I'd often end up somewhere in la-la land—not quite asleep and not quite awake, where thoughts blurred and I ended up just wasting time spinning my wheels on nonsense rather than doing anything truly productive.

The conveyor belt exercise would usually help me fall back asleep. This would last for a couple of hours before I'd find myself on my back, eyes popping wide open looking at the ceiling again, at 4:00 a.m. This time, I would usually have to go to the bathroom. Using mindfulness, I would get up slowly, noticing how my body felt cooler as I emerged from my cocoon of blankets. I would notice the feel of the floor as I touched each socked foot to it. I would slowly walk, step by step, from my bedroom to the bathroom, guided by the faint glow of little night-lights along the way. I would notice each step as I descended the staircase and the cool feel of the wooden banister as I slid my hand down it all along the way.

When I arrived in the bathroom, I wouldn't turn on the light. The automatic night-light sensed my arrival as I gently swung open the bathroom door, and I would notice lifting the lid to the commode, sitting down, feeling the cold seat, and then doing my business. I'd then sit there for a few more minutes, my eyes closed, and then I'd get up and wash my hands. I would notice the warm water on my skin, the scent and feel of the foamy, lathering lavender soap, and the feeling of the towel as I dried my hands. I would repeat my routine with the stairs, banister, and night-light lit hallways back to my bed. Sometimes, upon returning to bed, I would be able to close my eyes and repeat the conveyor belt exercise. When this wasn't effective, though, I noticed that. I reminded myself that it was very human of me to be frustrated about not being able to sleep. I extended compassion to myself—a very different approach to insomnia, right?

If after twenty minutes I was still wide awake (and no, I wasn't staring at or repeatedly looking at the clock, but I would tend to automatically look at it around the fifteen- to twenty-minute mark), I would make the choice to get up and out of bed, regardless of it being so early. At that point, I was making the mindful decision to go to my home office and do some work on the computer. Although I know that light from electronic devices only serves to stimulate us more, I had accepted that returning to sleep anytime soon didn't appear to be on the horizon. So rather than toss and turn, mumble, get angry, and spin my wheels on nonproductive long-winded thoughts, I would do some work. Sometimes just being up for an hour was enough to make me tired enough to get back to sleep. Sometimes not. Either way, I noticed my experience and did the best I could.

Can you relate to this real-world example? In what area of your life might you strategically apply what you've learned about the concepts of mindfulness and accepting reality from this DBT perspective?

Examining Your Experience Under a Mindfulness Microscope

Let's dive into some more skills that you can begin to use right away. It's time to begin enlisting your inner scientist by examining your experiences under a mindfulness microscope. It may sound a bit corny, or hey, it may appeal to you in the same way it does to me. I love learning about how our brains and nervous systems work, their anatomy, and why our brains and nervous systems react and respond in the ways that they do.

In those moments when I'm becoming emotionally dysregulated, it can be helpful to use the imagery of myself as an observer of my experience—like a scientist—because doing this keeps me from becoming completely enmeshed in and swept up and away by my thoughts and emotions. So give this visualization a try. Essentially, the goal of this skill is to get us looking at what's happening without completely identifying with it. For example, perhaps, like me, you sometimes suffer from anxiety attacks. Before learning to mindfully observe my emotions, *I am anxious* was quite a literal experience for me. I was the anxiety. I had no sense of separation: that I was the one *experiencing* the anxiety.

I was so intertwined with it that the intensity level of my experience of that emotion was astronomical. In the midst of such intensity, it is very difficult to think clearly or to have any hope that the emotion will ever end, which can lead to feeling desperate, which can lead to impulsive behaviors in an attempt to feel better, which can lead to regret, and then it just becomes a vicious cycle. Is this resonating with you? It's okay. Most of us were never taught to separate our thoughts and our emotions from the facts of the experience we are living in the present moment. DBT allows us to learn and practice these skills and reduce our emotional suffering.

Noticing what's happening within us and then putting words to our experience can be incredibly helpful. For example, while in the midst of an anxiety attack, observing my experience under the mindfulness microscope and then speaking aloud or to myself what I am noticing would take my mind-set from *I am anxious! Help! I'm freaking out! I can't take this! This is never going to end!*—a red alert to my nervous system that would perpetuate the anxiety attack—to this more mindful approach:

I am experiencing the emotion of anxiety.

I am noticing the thought that "This is never going to end." And it is just a thought, not a fact.

I am noticing that my heart is racing and that I'm short of breath.

These are normal physiological responses to anxiety, and they will pass.

I can notice them and trust they will pass.

Through this observation, I am giving my nervous system a chance to calm down so that this anxiety attack can end sooner.

In this moment, I will focus on my breath, slowing it down to an even pace.

I will choose to take care of myself and lie down and wait for the storm to pass, as it inevitably will.

You may now be thinking to yourself, *Yeah, right, Debbie! There is no way that I can get myself together enough in the midst of an anxiety attack and calmly speak to myself this way.* And, that's what I used to think, too. To be fair, in the midst of an anxiety or panic attack, it can be immensely difficult to tap into your inner voice of reason and redirect your attention, but I can tell you from personal experience that there will be opportunities. Even during an anxiety attack, there will be little glimmers of opening in which you can practice. If you pay attention, you will realize that you have a choice to be swept up in the suffering or to take hold of your mind and begin to comfort yourself emotionally and quell the physical upset triggered by the nervous system's attempt to protect you from a real or imagined fear or trigger. It's not easy. It took me a lot of practice, but to this day, I use this skill to keep anxiety, which inevitably makes its reappearance now and again, from emotionally hijacking me.

Real-World Activity:
Place a Slide Under the Microscope

What emotion do you find causes you the most hardship? Is it anger? Sadness? Anxiety? Recall an experience that recently evoked this emotion. If a similar situation were to present itself again in the near future, how might you use the mindfulness microscope to observe your experience without getting consumed by it? What might you say to yourself? Try working through the following example in your notebook. Fill in the blanks with your own responses, first naming the emotion that causes you the most hardship, followed by a thought that might accompany this emotion, and your physical responses, and so on. For example, if you were to feel social anxiety, you might think, *The whole group is interacting, and I'm so boring that no one is paying attention to me.* You might write that you feel a tightness in your stomach or clammy hands.

I am experiencing the emotion of _____.
(Name the emotion that causes you the most hardship.)

*I am noticing the thought "*_____,*" which is just a thought, and not necessarily a fact.*

I am noticing (physiological responses/body sensations), including

_____.

These are normal physiological responses to this emotion of _____ *and they will pass.*

I can notice them and trust they will pass.

Through this observation, I give my nervous system a chance to calm down, so that this episode can end sooner.

In this moment, I will focus on _____.
(Name some internal actions that will help you reduce the emotion, such as unclenching your fists if you are feeling anger or thinking about positive things if you are feeling sad, slowing down your breath if you are having anxiety, or letting go of tension in your jaw, shoulders, and neck and focusing on what others are saying if you are feeling social anxiety.)

I will choose to take care of myself by _____,
and will wait for the storm to pass, as it inevitably will.

Were you able to think of ways you could take care of yourself in the situation while waiting for the storm to pass? For example, if you were feeling social anxiety, you could say something like, *I will remind myself that no one can be the star of the conversation and center of attention all the time.* If you were unable to think of anything, don't worry. There are a number of ways to do this, and we will return to this topic again. For now, it's most important to concentrate your efforts on being an observer of your experience when you feel strong and difficult emotions. Being able to do this is a great first step.

Stay in the Lab, and Keep on Your Lab Coat

In order for this mindfulness practice to truly be effective, you must completely throw yourself into the experience at hand. For example, if I were using the above self-talk to mindfully observe and describe my experience of an anxiety attack, doing so while Googling "heart attacks" or "Am I going to faint?" would not be mindfully attending to the moment. I'd be diverting my attention in ways that would be counterproductive to my intention of sitting with my experience, allowing the emotion to run its course, and then getting on with my day in a more regulated manner. So, when working mindfully with an emotion, be sure to stay in the laboratory. Now is not the time to walk to the water cooler or to get back in your street clothes. When practicing mindfulness, put in 100 percent of your efforts, attention, and energy. This is how you will begin to see real and meaningful results.

Your Inner Judge and Jury

Okay, after all that fuss about staying in the lab, we're actually going to take a brief break to visit the courtroom of the mind. We all have an inner judge and jury, and unfortunately, we can't get out of this kind of jury duty. You know the old saying about how we are our own worst critics? This is often true. It's human to judge. As humans, we often even take it a step further to self-condemnation, a state that does little to help us stay emotionally regulated. Judging actually serves a purpose and is a shorthand of sorts when it comes to making decisions about whether something is good or bad, safe or unsafe, trustworthy or untrustworthy, healthy or unhealthy, and so on. The problem with judgments is that it can be very easy to mistake them for facts when often they are only our opinions. Treating judgments as facts has caused me a world of emotional pain over the years. Is this a problem for you too? The key to sparing ourselves from this kind of pain is to learn how to identify and reduce judgments that have no value for us.

Many people with BPD have unrealistic expectations of perfection. Sometimes this is outwardly directed. We may be gravely disappointed and lose all faith in someone we previously admired, because she messed up on one little thing. Maybe your hairdresser forgot to write down your appointment, and you showed up to find out that you had to wait another week to get your blowout. Maybe a friend is unable to keep the plans the two of you made for dinner because he has to work late. While people who aren't emotionally sensitive can usually categorize these types of incidents in the "Oh, well, things happen" category and then adjust their plans accordingly, for those of us with BPD traits, these types of situations can come off as being, at some level, intentional slights and cause us deep emotional pain, even if they are actually not the offending party's fault.

At the more extreme level, which isn't unusual when you're dealing with lots of emotional dysregulation, these perceived slights may be internalized as a form of rejection and abandonment, which can lead to even more despair. It can be really painful to be in this particular mental space, so it makes sense to me that when we are hurt, we sometimes judge. That way, we can put the blame on someone or something else and make them "wrong" and us "right." It's a defense mechanism to reduce the hurt. If that person is a jerk because she forgot to write me down or he's self-absorbed because he's canceling our dinner plans, I don't have to focus too much on the fact that I feel disappointed, sad, and maybe even disrespected, all of which are difficult emotional states to bear when you are sensitive.

EXAMINING SELF-JUDGMENT

The other way that judgments often come up for us is when we make judgments about ourselves. If we hold others to very high standards, we also tend to have even higher expectations for ourselves. I grew up in a household where if I upset my father, there was a price to pay. A scary price. The abuse still haunts me to this day. I had to learn, as best as I could, to survive under those circumstances and learn to please my father to avoid his wrath. When I was in grade school, if I didn't get all As, I was spanked. I came home one time from school, terrified of what was to come.

You bet your bippy that, from that point on, I became someone who excelled academically. I was made to fear imperfection in this area, and as you can imagine, this striving for perfection carried over to other areas of my life. It carried over to my body image, and I struggled on and off, in secret, with undiagnosed anorexia for much of my childhood and adolescence. Sadly, my recollections are far from rare. I hear such accounts from peers around the world who now have BPD or who identify as severely emotionally sensitive.

Even though many of us have gone on to find some healing and to seek out and begin practicing healthier behaviors, we still find perfectionism to be a major issue and source of suffering in our lives. And what is perfectionism really? It's judging yourself against an unrealistic expectation: being perfect. It is knowing that being perfect is unrealistic but feeling driven and compelled to strive for it anyway. It's holding yourself to standards that you'd probably never truly expect from anyone else. You know this from a place of inner wisdom, but your intense emotions say, *Don't ease up. You'll lose everything,* or some other scary, threatening, untruthful catastrophic message.

We are essentially making judgments all day long, and much of this is rooted in our past pain and experiences. We judge things like the weather ... how the person next to us in the coffee shop looks ... how our neighbors are raising their children ... how our family members are living their lives ... that we made a mistake, be it minor or major. Again, the main problem with judgments from a DBT perspective is that we all too often believe our judgments to be facts, when this is not always the case, which leads to lots of unnecessary suffering.

MAKING JUDGMENTS USEFUL

Stating your dismay with something in the form of a judgment gives you very little room to move and shift and overcome the issue that's troubling you. It leaves you stuck. For example, let's say you consider yourself to be a "bad employee." That doesn't give you or anyone you may be reaching out to about the problem sufficient information to work on changing the problem or your concern. To make judgments useful, we must be willing to pull out our microscopes again and examine them more closely.

Most importantly, we want to rewrite our judgments in a way that identifies the consequences of the upsetting matter, or whatever upset us in the first place and caused us to make the judgment. I'll give you a couple of before-and-after examples and then ask you to try doing this on your own.

Judgment: *I'm a bad employee.*

Consequences: *Sometimes, due to depression, I am not 100 percent focused on my tasks, so my productivity drops, and when this happens, my boss expresses disappointment in me. This makes me feel ashamed, more depressed, and like hurting myself.*

See the difference? In the original judgment you are stuck. But with the rewrite you have something to work with! You can think about ways to manage better at work when you are depressed, how to deal with your boss's reaction—as well as identify how much of your perception of her reaction is based on your thoughts and assumptions and how much of your perception is fact-based—and work on skillful strategies for coping with difficult emotions that may arise when you're feeling depressed and your work is impacted. Here's another example:

Judgment: *Sondra is a total jerk.*

Consequences: *Sondra canceled our plans at the last minute. I was really looking forward to our time together* *and am feeling disappointed, sad, and, to be honest, angry. I'm not sure if it's a fact or just my thoughts, but I think she was being rude and inconsiderate. She should know how easily I get upset.*

Okay, again in this example, simply calling Sondra, someone let's say you've been friends with for a while now and who is usually a reliable person, a "total jerk" leaves you stuck. In this case, the rewrite of the judgment started out from a mindful perspective, but did you notice a divergence into yet another judgment? Let's break it down. Acknowledging the fact that Sondra canceled plans at the last minute is nonjudgmental. Next, acknowledging how you feel as a result of the disappointment is also being nonjudgmental. It's an assessment of your experience. Your inner wisdom continues into the next sentence with the mindful observation that you realize that you may be believing your judgmental thought that Sondra is rude and inconsiderate. And then lastly comes the *should-statement*. I remember once hearing some advice not to "should all over" ourselves and that we must be careful that we're not "shoulding" on other people (Bassett 2006).

When you see or hear or say the word "should," you know you're dealing with a judgment. In this case, you're saying that Sondra should know how sensitive you are (and maybe she does), but you're also implying that she knew this and deliberately hurt you anyway. You can see how believing that judgments are facts, essentially assuming that they are true, can lead to unnecessary suffering. So, even when you think you're ready to take the judgment slide off of the microscope, consider reflecting, reviewing, and revising your rewrite until you are certain that you have written only about observable facts and have not added an opinion to the facts. You could still acknowledge that you think that Sondra should know how sensitive you are and that she should know better, but to do so mindfully would be to rephrase it as "I am *having a thought* that Sondra should know better."

Real-World Activity:
Examining Your Judgment

Now it's your turn. Grab your notebook, and think of something you judged today or recently. Without censoring yourself, write down the judgment exactly how it occurred to you and how you said it to yourself or out loud. Then, before even doing your rewrite, ask yourself if your judgment leaves you anywhere to go to improve or remedy the situation. If it's a true judgment, it does not. Next, list the following:

- *What about this situation triggered me to feel an emotion?*

- *What emotions did I feel or am I feeling?*

- *What are the consequences of the situation?*

Now rewrite your judgment identifying the consequences of the upsetting situation, or whatever caused you to make the judgment to begin with. After you are done, put your rewrite back under the microscope and look for any possible judgments that may be still lingering. Do another rewrite if needed.

How are you feeling about your judgment now? Do you see any opportunities for working on resolving the issue that has been troubling you?

Another way to reduce judgments is to count them as they occur throughout the day. You can find an app for your phone, or if you want to go old-school, carry around a small notepad and pen or one of those clickers they use to keep score for elementary school sports. Every time you notice a judgment during the day, be it about yourself, someone else, or circumstances, log it. Then at the end of each day, notice how many judgments you've had. As you continue to learn and practice mindfulness and to rewrite your judgments, notice if their number begins to go down. Paying attention to them usually causes this happen.

Doing What Works for the Situation

Whether you're working on reducing your judgments, becoming more mindfully aware of your experience from moment to moment, or practicing any other DBT skill, really, the objective is to do what works in the situation. What actually works is going to be different from one situation to the next and will depend on your short- and long-term goals. The question to ask yourself in any given situation is, *If I choose this action or behavior, is the outcome likely to keep me on track with meeting the goals I am working so hard to reach? Will it likely be effective?* Then choose how to behave based on how badly you want to stay on track with achieving your goals.

Let's say that you've been working on the goal of getting your needs met by being assertive. You find yourself in a situation where you ask for assistance, and the person on the other end of the conversation is not being very cooperative. Being effective at accomplishing your goal in such a situation can be challenging but doable. I'll share a technical nightmare I dealt with concerning my company website. I called our hosting company for assistance and ended up on hold for a good forty-five minutes. When the tech support guy finally got on the phone, I explained the situation.

Although I was patting myself on the back for waiting so patiently and believed I was doing an excellent job of carefully describing the issues I was facing, his responses indicated that he didn't quite understand what I was experiencing, which began to frustrate me. I kept my cool and explained again. When it finally seemed as if he understood, he told me that there was nothing that could be done to fix the issues I was reporting. I thought he also sounded a little cocky and dismissive. In the past, in a situation like this, I would become quite irate. I would get rude with the technical support person. I would make demands. As a result of this behavior, as you can imagine, the human being on the other end of the line was very often not too willing to help me further. Either he would reiterate that there was nothing he could do or I'd be suddenly disconnected from the line.

I didn't want either of these things to happen on this call. Remember, my objective in this situation was to effectively meet my goal of getting my website fixed by being assertive. I knew that to achieve this goal, I had to make different choices than I'd made in the past. I began with some small talk with the rep, saying things like, "Wow. The hold time is long today. You guys must be inundated over there." This seemed to defuse the situation and get him to open up a little. My intention was to make a meaningful connection with him and get him to see that I understood that he's a human being dealing with stress on his end, too. I then expressed to him that my business was missing out on traffic because of my website issues, I was really concerned, and that it seemed like my issue was unusual. I asked if perhaps my call needed to be transferred to a supervisor.

Notice that I didn't threaten or insult him, "You don't know what you're doing. Put your supervisor on the line, you incompetent idiot!" That would have been the old Debbie, who would have been accidentally disconnected. This time, I chose my words carefully and behaved much more empathetically, expressing that I simply needed a solution. The rep's tone changed. He slowed down. He offered to look at more things to try to determine what was happening. In doing this, he discovered some issues contributing to my problem and made some recommendations that ultimately helped. I didn't have to speak to a supervisor after all, nor did I need to call back and wait another forty-five minutes to speak to someone new. My issue was resolved. So, despite the intense feelings of frustration, annoyance, and helplessness that I felt at the onset of the call, and despite urges that arose to do some very unskillful things in response, keeping mindful of my goals in the situation helped me to accomplish what I needed in that moment. I did what worked. I chose behaviors that were effective for the situation.

Sometimes my students ask how to discern whether you're actually manipulating someone or you're just being skillful in your attempt to be effective in an interaction. In the situation with the rep, was I being phony or manipulating him by making small talk and trying to convey that I understood that he's human and dealing with pressures, too? Well, I recall that it certainly was difficult for me to muster up some compassion for him in the midst of my frustration and anxiety, but doing so was, in fact, skillful and not manipulative.

My rule of thumb is to ask myself how I feel during and after an interaction. Lying, exaggerating, or being intimidating to get what you want would fall under being manipulative. Adjusting your strategy when you have a need, by acknowledging the other person's perspective and being willing to give a little or show empathy, is a skillful approach. It's about intention. I'll also point out that sometimes, no matter how well you are applying these skills, you may not get what you want. Coping effectively with the disappointment of such an outcome takes another set of skills to manage the emotions that can arise. We will go more into this in chapter 4.

Conscious Redirection of the Mind

The next mindfulness skill is conscious redirection of the mind. You're going to practice further strengthening your mindfulness muscle and refocusing your attention to where you want it to be in any given moment. In today's world of website woes and our always-on tech-centric society, with screens of all sizes constantly competing for our attention, we actually have plenty of opportunities to practice this skill every day. An excellent way to begin to practice this skill is to start observing your urges to check and use your cell phone and then sometimes choose to redirect your attention to do something else instead, such as having a conversation, meditating, reading, going for a walk, or noticing your surroundings.

With time and practice, you'll eventually build confidence in your ability to shift your attention elsewhere in other situations in life when doing so can be really helpful. This could be when you notice you're getting caught up in worry thoughts, those ruminations about the past and future that get you, in the most extreme of cases, caught up in dissociative states and feeling completely disconnected from what's happening in the moment. In these situations, you'll be able to redirect your mind to where you want it to be.

Real-World Activity:
Disconnect to Reconnect

The next time you're waiting in line or are in another typical situation where you have the urge to pull out your phone, consider choosing to notice that urge, and rather than giving in immediately, redirect your focus to something else. Choose to be mindfully aware of what you can notice through each of your senses. Look for opportunities to connect with other people or animals or the environment in real time. Look around and consider what you might have missed if you had turned to your phone in this moment. See people. See nature. Hear sounds. Touch something. Notice how you feel. See how long you can stick with it before taking out and using your phone. Jot down your experiences in your notebook.

Something that can support your effort as you're working on this skill is disabling all nonessential pop-up notifications and sound alerts. I no longer get an alert on my cell phone every time someone tweets me or likes my posts. These were just more unnecessary pulls on my attention from the present moment. When I want to get an update on what's happening online, I can open the apps or log in at my computer and devote some time to mindfully reviewing those things. You can do the same.

As you get better and better at consciously redirecting your mind, using your cell phone urges for practice, you may begin to notice that you're feeling better equipped to practice this mindfulness skill in other situations. You may want to come up with a game plan for specific situations and challenging moments in which you can begin applying this technique. As with reaching for the cell phone or not, you'll have the option to notice urges to engage with upsetting thoughts and the ability to choose to redirect your attention to something more constructive, such as problem solving, asking for support, or distracting yourself with other things.

Accepting Reality to Reduce Suffering

The next skill to practice is choosing to accept reality. Accepting reality is easy when life is going the way we want it to and we aren't experiencing an upset or challenge, but painful moments, like feeling slighted, not getting something we desire, or feeling alone and scared, present us with opportunities to practice accepting reality and reduce our emotional suffering. As mentioned earlier, pain is inevitable, but suffering is optional. What does this really mean? Some things in life are incredibly difficult to accept because facing and accepting them causes emotional pain. Take the case of someone accepting that a spouse has been cheating. While denying it and pretending it isn't happening might seem a lot easier and less painful, accepting reality puts the person in a position of power to then take action to change her circumstances. Staying in denial and not accepting reality keeps us stuck and suffering, whether it's in an unhealthy relationship, a toxic work environment, or not getting the help we need for mental health issues.

The paradox is that only through being willing to initially accept a situation as it is in this moment can we take any action to change our circumstances. This may sound a bit strange or counterintuitive at first, so let me explain. For many years, I was quite unconscious of the patterns that were holding me back in life, including in the context of intimate relationships. In my late teens and into my twenties, when my former partner would make comments to suggest that I might not be thinking clearly or that I seemed emotionally unstable, I was not at all receptive. I became defensive and quite aggressive in response to his suggestions. It was only when I was able to acknowledge that there might be some truth in his "accusations" that I realized I did need help and that I could begin to change and become a better partner.

At that point, I had to radically accept where I was in my life. I had to accept the reality that, at that moment in time, I was a broken person who didn't have the skills needed to be a healthy half of a romantic relationship. I had unresolved past trauma. I had an incredibly intense fear of being rejected and abandoned. If I had continued to deny that I had any issues with being in an intimate relationship—and stayed convinced that my partner was the one with the problem, and I had nothing to change—I would have remained stuck in a place where I was unable to have a healthy relationship. Only by accepting reality could I begin to explore options that would help me change that reality and break free from the drama I was unintentionally creating within and all around me.

One of those inspirational image quotes came up on my Facebook feed recently from author Doreen Virtue: "Where there is drama, there is unresolved trauma." I believe this is true not only for me but also for so many who are behaving outwardly in dysfunctional ways and having difficulty accepting reality in painful moments. Denying the reality of unresolved, unhealed pain and trauma is often the driving force. (It's important to note that accepting that we have experienced past trauma that's affecting us now doesn't mean we are letting someone who violated us off the hook. We are just admitting or acknowledging the reality that the trauma occurred. There's a big difference.)

But when it comes to accepting reality, we are not limited to accepting events that are extreme or traumatic. Things come up on a daily basis that, without our acceptance, can turn into sources of suffering. It's raining and you had a big picnic party planned. Perhaps you didn't get that job you were hoping for. Someone you have feelings for has not returned them. Accepting something doesn't necessarily mean that you like, agree with, or approve of the circumstances. It means you are using your inner wisdom to simply acknowledge the reality, as it is, in that moment—that something is or was real, that it is happening or has happened. You might also call acceptance, "Reality Acknowledgement."

Here are some examples of how to do this in the above scenarios:

Acceptance: *I didn't get that job, and as a result, I'm feeling down and a bit hopeless.*

As opposed to *It's not fair that I didn't get that job … or … Those people are idiots for not hiring me … or … I'll never get another opportunity like this.* These responses are judgments or predictions rather than accepting reality.

Acceptance: *I really have intense feelings for Gabriel, but he doesn't feel the same way. I feel hurt and worried I'll never feel this way about anyone else again and will stay alone forever.*

As opposed to *There must be something I can do to change his mind … or … If I just keep trying to convince him of how wonderful we'd be together, he'd see the light … or … I'll never feel this way again and will be alone forever!* Notice that last sentence. What distinguishes it from the earlier accepting-reality thought? The same worries are mentioned, but instead of noticing them as worry thoughts, they are stated as facts.

Acceptance: *It's raining out, so now I have to change my plans for the picnic. I feel angry and disappointed. So much work went into this, and a lot of people have been looking forward to it, including me.*

As opposed to *This isn't fair! … or … Bad things always happen to me. Why today?*

Think about how you might feel after each of these events had you gone the radical acceptance–reality acknowledgment route versus the nonacceptance (resistance, denial, or complaining) route.

Noticing Opportunities for Practice

Last but not least, when it comes to practicing mindfulness, be aware that as you become equipped with skills, you will notice more and more opportunities to use them. There will also be times when you're feeling stuck and stubborn and unwilling to use your skills even though you now have them at your disposal. This can happen for many reasons, including believing it's more important to be right than to be effective. This can be because impulse control is still an issue.

You may have additional reasons or excuses when the time comes—that fork in the road where you have to decide if you're going to go down the old road of self-sabotage, self-destruction, and unskillfulness or if you will choose the newly paved, much more rewarding DBT Path (the powerful visual that has had so much meaning for me that it helped me name my online school!). You will need to make this choice over and over again. To this day, I must do the same.

The good news is that the more we choose our skills over our old behaviors, the more this choice gets reinforced in our brain, and the more natural and easier it is to choose this path in the future. I know this from personal experience. The skills, for the most part, are interwoven throughout my day. During times of stress or emotional distress, I notice that I have to be more mindful to actively choose to be skillful, and I'm not successful all the time. But, most of the time, I manage to make the choice that is most effective and end up practicing the DBT skills to avoid unnecessary suffering and to keep me moving toward and achieving and maintaining my goals. The same will be possible for you.

This is the challenge. Notice those forks in the road. Applaud yourself for the times when you choose to be skillful, and mindfully reflect on what happens when you end up choosing the nonskillful road. Don't judge yourself. Consider journaling the reasons that led to either choice, so you can reinforce your skillful behavior choices and reduce and eliminate your nonskillful choices. As time goes on, if you stay committed and keep working at it, you'll likely notice yourself tapping into your own inner wisdom a lot more often, feeling more balanced, and knowing you are truly working on building the life you want to live.

You now have the major foundation of DBT mindfulness under your belt with an understanding of some skills and ideas for immediate practice. As you read on and learn more, refer back to this chapter frequently. As I mentioned earlier, this section is the longest in the book for a reason. It is your reference section. When you're having difficulty putting a particular skill into action, refer back here to work on bringing the quality of mindfulness that's needed to increase your chances of success.

Again, mindfulness truly is the great foundation for all of the other DBT skills, so it's important that we started with it first.

Next, you'll begin learning how to cope more effectively with distress, particularly in moments and in situations that are causing you stress but that have no immediate remedy or solution. We must learn to mindfully tolerate such distress to avoid self-sabotaging and causing ourselves greater emotional suffering. So, are you ready? Here we go.

Chapter 2

Coping Effectively
with Distress

When we feel intense anxiety or emotional pain in response to upsetting events, we're experiencing emotional distress. Being at the mercy of distress, not knowing how to be skillful when something upsets us, leaves us vulnerable to progressively spiraling out of control and into the self-sabotaging behaviors that we are working so hard to avoid. Learning how to tolerate distress and cope in upsetting situations is essential for handling life's ups and downs and avoiding making already difficult situations worse. By practicing coping effectively, taking actions to reduce your distress level and suffering, you can intervene on your own behalf and break this vicious cycle. This chapter will introduce some skills that are designed to help you do just this.

Tolerating Distress Takes Practice

For those of us who routinely experience emotional dysregulation, skillfully tolerating distress often doesn't come naturally.

We must learn how to do it. We must practice it. Through a willingness to learn and master these skills to the best of our ability, we can set ourselves up to function better in this world. That's pretty awesome when you think about it. It's not too late for us. Even as adults, we can learn these skills and change our lives so that they look more like what we desire. We can move forward, achieve goals, and break the cycle of self-sabotage in which we never make any progress.

We can learn to accept the reality that we cannot completely avoid upsetting circumstances and situations. We can learn to accept and deal with the fact that some issues can't be resolved as quickly as we'd like and that we can find ways to skillfully wait things out. Difficult situations are precisely the times when we can call upon and practice tolerating distress so that we don't make matters worse. The acceptance part will largely come from knowing that we are equipped with skills to handle such situations and we can make healthy choices.

Unskillful choices, such as drinking, using drugs, or reckless spending, may soothe us and quell our emotional pain momentarily but are harmful in both the short run and the long run. Each of these behaviors brings its own set of consequences, and then we're left with even more to deal with, needing to engage in damage control to clean up the new messes we've created, compounding the original problem. We must begin learning and choosing new courses of action, and we do this one new skillful decision at a time. The more you practice tolerating distress, the more natural it will become. When you take a chance and give some of these effective strategies a try, you might even surprise yourself. The payoff of knowing that you haven't made matters worse is worth it, in and of itself, and this sense of gratification serves to reinforce future skillful choices, bringing you closer to your goals and values.

As you're practicing the art and science of skillfully tolerating distress, the ultimate rule is this: if you're facing a stressful situation that can be fixed or resolved, your first line of defense is to try problem solving to fix or resolve it. If the situation cannot be fixed or resolved in that moment, and you want to get through it without making matters worse by creating more problems for yourself, practice skillfully tolerating the distress. You can practice tolerating distress by keeping your cool in such everyday situations as being stuck in traffic and late for work, awaiting medical tests that may have a scary outcome, or waiting to hear back from someone you've been unable to reach. In each of these situations, there is nothing you can do to change the situation: you can't speed up traffic, you can't hurry the lab to get your test results any sooner, and you can't reach someone who is out of cell phone range. In each situation, the goal is to find a way to manage your response so that you can reduce unnecessary suffering and tolerate the moment. The moment will pass. You just have to survive it intact.

Now, believe me, I know all too well that when we're at the height of emotional distress, the waiting period for an answer or an outcome, or until we think things might be less stressful, can feel like it might last forever. Like a slow, taunting eternity.

In order to not turn to destructive behaviors for immediate comfort in a moment of desperation and despair, we must deliberately and repeatedly remind ourselves that the stressful situation is indeed temporary—it is not going to last forever—and that we only have to tolerate it one moment at a time. In the example of waiting on medical test results, for example, you could tell yourself, *The doctor said the results will be in on Monday. It's Thursday today. I can get through three more days. Here's how I'll tolerate the distress in the meantime* ...

If three days seems too daunting, you can break down your distress tolerance goals into even smaller time intervals, to where you are working on getting through each day, hour by hour and even minute by minute, until the distress goes down to a level where it no longer consumes you and will no longer be a catalyst for unmindful, unskillful behaviors.

Real-World Example: Road Rage

Getting stuck behind a slow driver is a great opportunity for practicing tolerating distress. Maybe this particular scenario has triggered you to experience distress in the past, and getting stuck behind a slow driver is something that will inevitably happen again—even as soon as the next time you head somewhere in your car. Choosing to tolerate distress in this scenario can make all the difference in how you feel after the experience and whether you compound or reduce your problems and distress.

So imagine this: there you are, minding your own business, just trying to make it to your first day at a new job, and you are stuck behind a slow driver. You are expected to be at your destination in twenty minutes, and your GPS shows that you have thirty-two minutes to go before you can expect to arrive. You feel your blood boiling. Your heart is racing. Your hands are getting sweaty. Why is this jackass going so slow in front of you on a two-way road that doesn't allow for passing? Maybe he has nowhere to go, but you do, and you're rapidly losing your patience and your cool.

Even though it's broad daylight, you begin flashing your headlights and your high beams in the hopes that this clueless driver will get the hint. He doesn't. It's as if he were in his own little bubble, unaware of his surroundings or your frantic efforts to get his attention. *Move … over!!!* Miles later, and he's still going five miles below the posted speed limit, pushing your estimated time of arrival out even further. Sure, you could respond by pulling over and calling the person you're meeting to let her know you're running late (problem solving) and by taking a break and doing some deep breathing (self-care), but neither of these things occurs to you, or even if it does, your anger takes over and trumps any such rational thinking.

Your emotional distress escalates, and you're now revving the engine and riding dangerously close to the bumper of the slow driver in front of you, when, uh oh … a police officer is coming down the road in the opposite direction. You hope he didn't notice but realize there's no way he couldn't have. Within minutes, there are flashing lights behind you. You are being pulled over and now are going to be so late and have additional consequences to deal with, including paying a costly ticket and perhaps an increase on your insurance premium.

I've been there. I used to behave like a wild animal when I was stuck behind a slow driver and needed to be somewhere on time. Perhaps this resonates with you because you've experienced your own share of frustration in driving situations and may even have experienced road rage in some of the same ways that I have. With DBT skills specifically designed for tolerating distress (such as the distress of being behind a clueless, slow driver), I have learned that there is absolutely no point in getting myself worked up that way. It's useless! Swearing, honking my horn, flashing lights, tailgating, and yelling didn't get me to my destination any faster than being skillful, remaining calm, and making the best of an upsetting, inconvenient situation would have gotten me, but it did upset my nervous system and cause me to feel even more dysregulated.

Getting stressed gets your heart and breathing rates up and your adrenaline flowing, which will make you feel worse both physically and mentally. Losing your cool can lead to behaving in ways that compromise your self-respect, causing you to feel shame or guilt. Believe me, I didn't like myself very much when I had calmed down and thought about how I might have scared the driver in front of me, or the shame I felt when interacting with a police officer about my behavior. The consequences of compromising your self-respect and feeling shame or guilt suck, and they only add to your initial distress and multiply it. To avoid or reduce this unnecessary suffering, the very first step in distress-provoking situations is to call upon your newly learned mindfulness skills.

Step Back from the Situation

The first step is to notice what you can about the situation and the thoughts you're having in response to it. Use some self-coaching to remind yourself that the problem is beyond your control (something that is often very difficult to accept and tolerate, but once you do, it makes a world of difference). Perhaps something like *This guy either doesn't see me trying to get his attention or is not willing to go any faster. I'm pissed, but clearly there's nothing I can do about either of those things.* Channel your inner wisdom to remind yourself that others, especially those whom you may be concerned about upsetting due to possibly being late, have likely also been in a similar situation and will hopefully understand. You can pull over when it's safe to do so and call them. When you're stuck behind a slow driver, that's the reality you're working with. Most people will understand.

Acknowledge your fears and what is driving (ah, yes, pun intended) the intense emotion. For example, perhaps you can identify that the reason you're getting so worked up is that you're afraid of being late to work. Our thoughts can quickly jump from *This slow traffic sucks!* to *I'm going to lose my job and be homeless on the street!* in a catastrophic flash. The problem with this reaction is that we're not using mindfulness to slow down the jump in thoughts, and we begin distressing and behaving as if the feared thought were already true. Unhealthy and reckless behaviors, like dangerous driving, follow suit. We're not taking the time to notice our thoughts. We're reacting to them instead. This is when we need to begin to intervene, first with mindfulness skills and then with tolerating distress, to learn to stay in and get through just *this* moment, not a scary scene playing out in our head of what more could go wrong.

Distract Yourself Mindfully

Tolerating distress in this particular example may come in the form of mindfully distracting yourself from the upsetting issue. Something that works for many people while driving is to turn on some good music on the radio. Sometimes I opt for an interesting talk-radio show that is engaging and gets my mind off of my tension and worries. If you're someone who finds music or the sound of people speaking to be soothing, this choice will allow you to self-soothe through sound. The bottom line is that while distracting yourself won't get you to your destination any faster, this can most definitely help keep you from losing control and creating suffering for yourself in the form of severe dysregulation. It's worth it!

You may be surprised at how effective seemingly very simple strategies, such as turning on the radio, can be at helping you feel more balanced and in control of your emotions. Our nervous systems are complex, and the messages we send to it matter. Keep practicing to learn which skills and strategies are most effective for you in different scenarios. You may also realize that you have been using some of these skills in your life already. For example, you may have always intuitively turned on music to help you calm down or made yourself warm tea to help you feel comforted when stressed out at home. As you continue to learn new skills and recognize ones that you're already using, you can refine them and increase your ability to make healthier choices more often to cope more effectively with emotional distress.

Show Self-Compassion

One of the things that surprised me about DBT and that my students also often comment on is how people who don't have emotional dysregulation or sensitivity issues seem to know and use these skills pretty automatically most of the time. They don't have to think things through like we do. Instead of behaving impulsively or in unhealthy ways when they're upset, they've developed the habit of being skillful. They may not understand why we have such a hard time getting it. When sharing what I was learning in DBT early on, I even had loved ones saying, "Well, that's just common sense," a comment that can come off as really degrading to people for whom these skills are not second nature and who didn't learn them as children. The great thing is that DBT uses what's called a *skills deficit model*. There is an assumption that many of us with BPD, for myriad reasons, didn't acquire these skills as children. Fortunately, we can learn and integrate them into our lives now!

Perhaps you've been in a similar conversation. It's difficult to not take a comment like this as an insult, but you need to do your best to have compassion for yourself as you work on learning and integrating these skills into your life. As emotionally sensitive people, we are not among the common anyway. We are tasked with lovingly and patiently teaching ourselves these skills as adults, and we can and do make positive differences in our lives by doing so—one step at a time, one practice at a time, one skillful distraction at a time—to prevent ourselves from making things worse. It is never too late to learn how to skillfully distract from our emotional pain.

Skillful Distraction vs. Avoidance

There is a difference between skillfully distracting yourself from emotional pain and avoiding emotional pain. The less skillful act of avoidance causes more problems in the long run. Because we avoid our feelings in an unmindful way while trying to dull and deny our emotional pain, we often end up engaging in harmful behaviors that do not serve us. In contrast, when we skillfully distract ourselves from our painful emotions, we are still conscious that the emotionally triggering event has occurred. We don't try to deny it and pretend that everything is hunky-dory. We acknowledge that we have a right to have our emotions and that we are only human. From this perspective, we then deliberately choose to manage our distress by pushing away our thoughts for a short period of time. We realize that our emotional distress in this moment is not serving us and not bringing us closer to our personal goals, and so we mindfully engage in activities and practices that allow us to take the focus off of the pain.

The purpose of distracting mindfully from pain is to keep us from becoming overwhelmed by something that can't be resolved, so we don't feel helpless, desperate for relief, and act out in impulsive ways that we'll later regret. Avoidance is often one of the ways that we cope with distress before we learn how to do something more constructive. This makes sense. If something hurts, we want to avoid it. If we touch the hot stove when we are little, it burns and hurts, so we learn to never touch it when it's hot again. As emotionally sensitive adults, we've learned that if something hurts emotionally, it's best to suppress it, deny it, and numb the pain however we can. This can come in the form of self-harm, drinking, using drugs, taking more or less of a prescription medication, having sex with strangers, spending tons of money foolishly, driving recklessly, and other self-destructive behaviors. Experiencing and enduring emotional distress does not feel like a viable option when you lack the skills to manage it. Instead, the urge is to stop it. Fast.

I certainly felt that way. Fortunately, over time, practicing distress management has worked like an emotional inoculation to allow me to experience even painful emotions without becoming completely derailed, going into crying spells, and ending up suicidal, all of which used to happen quite regularly. I have the same hope for you. So, as much as an inoculation may sound terrifying, it's time to get brave, roll up that sleeve, and begin to experience tiny doses of tolerating distress. I am delighted when my students report the feelings of success, accomplishment, and pride that occur when they are able to handle things that would previously have caused them to create problems in their relationships, work, and at school. My hope is that you too will begin to notice small changes that bring you a sense of pride and accomplishment. This isn't easy work, but it's worth it. Let's look at some skills you can begin practicing today.

Setting Aside Thoughts for a Time

Choosing to put aside certain distressing thoughts for a time is a skillful way to cope, whereas dwelling on upsetting thoughts and staying stuck in a ruminating (repetitive, obsessive) unproductive state leads to more distress and then to undesired behaviors. It does us no good, when we are trying to sleep, work, or even enjoy a good television program or otherwise relax, to be consumed with worry thoughts about an event that we can do nothing to solve in that moment.

Setting aside thoughts can be very effective at helping us get unstuck from worries that we can't solve, even if it's just for a little bit. We can experience that period of time with less suffering. Sometimes when I am ruminating, stuck in repetitive, obsessive thinking, I will practice imagining putting those thoughts onto a piece of paper and tucking it away in a little lockbox. I then envision myself placing that lockbox on the top shelf of a very high bookcase that I cannot easily access. Using imagery allows us to mindfully and temporarily push away thoughts that are not serving us. This simple exercise can be really helpful in convincing the mind that it's okay to let go for a little while.

Real-World Activity:
Consciously Pushing Away Distressing Thoughts

Do you have a situation you can practice with right now? Is there a nagging worry thought that is persisting even though you can't solve the problem right now? It's okay if you can't identify something in this moment. Just jot down this page number and topic, so you can quickly turn to it the next time a situation presents itself. If you're ready, let's begin!

What imagery works best for you? Placing this thought …

- on a high bookshelf?

- in a box or chest by the road?

- on a leaf floating down the river?

- on a cloud drifting by?

- something else?

Allow yourself the opportunity to imagine step-by-step setting aside the thought in the manner of your choosing. Notice how you feel and if you're able to release the distressing thought, even if just for a short amount of time, noting that you will revisit the issue when you're feeling better able to do so.

I do want to address a potential important concern before moving on from this skill. As someone who has experienced trauma and knows that in my younger years I understandably tried to deny it (*That never happened ... I couldn't handle it if it did, so it never happened ...*), this type of thought pushing might feel like more of the same. It is not. Please notice the important distinction here that we are not denying that something upsetting is happening or has happened. In fact, we are wholeheartedly acknowledging that it is happening or has happened. We then imagine setting it aside for a short period to give us some needed space until we feel better equipped to handle it. This could be when problem solving becomes an option or when we can process the event with outside support.

Put on Your Random-Acts-of-Kindness Hat

The previous exercise allows us to go inward into our imagination to cope effectively with distress and to experience the benefit of reduced suffering. There are other ways to cope that can benefit not only us but also those around us. Sometimes when we are feeling bad, the last thing we'd think to do is to put that pain on hold to help someone else, but this can actually be an incredibly powerful, effective, and rewarding skill. Contributing to the happiness of others has a twofold reward: we distract ourselves by getting outside of our own head and problems, focusing on how we can help someone else, and we inevitably feel joy at the other person's expression of appreciation. Even if you prefer to do your random acts of kindness in secret, you will experience the personal satisfaction of knowing you have done something kind.

I don't really believe it's possible to engage in an altruistic act, where we're doing something to benefit someone or something else, and gain absolutely nothing in return—and that's okay! It's partly why this skill works. The benefactor of an animal shelter who makes an anonymous million-dollar donation feels a sense of warmth in her heart, knowing how far that money will stretch to help animals in desperate need. (She'll also probably receive the reward of a major tax benefit.) It's perfectly human to feel joy when you do something kind for someone or something else, and this doesn't make your act of kindness selfish, cause it to have any less impact, or make it any less effective at helping you tolerate your distress. In fact, I think that in addition to distracting yourself by helping others, the emotional payoff also really helps. Here's another example that might be more realistic for most of us than making a million-dollar donation.

I was super stressed out the other day while running some errands. Earlier that morning, I had slipped in my socks and fallen down some steps, so my whole body was sore. My cell phone battery was dying, and I knew I needed to buy a new battery or a new phone. It was extremely hot outside, and I was tired. I really didn't feel like dealing with anything. I wanted to just go back home and go to sleep, but I was about forty-five minutes away from my place at this point. All of these things combined had me feeling quite grumpy.

I knew that problem solving would help, but first I needed to skillfully tolerate the distress I was feeling. Just then, as I was approaching the door of my cell phone provider, I saw a teeny tiny dog running around loose. I chased after him, calling to him somewhat frantically, because he was heading in the direction of a very busy street. As I did so, a homeless person came around the corner. He stared at me. At that moment, I realized that the dog was his. I let him know that I'd thought the dog was on his own. His response was, "Do you have fifty cents, so my dog can eat?"

My heart went out to both of them. I asked about whether he needed a leash, and he said, "No, she stays with me," which both concerned me and further warmed my heart. I reached into my purse but was fumbling because I was also carrying a large cup of coffee in my other hand. He offered to hold the cup. Now I'm a bit of a germophobe, but I thanked him and handed him the cup. I gave him some money, he handed back my cup, and we parted ways. Afterward, with my specialty coffee drink in one hand and my smart phone that was about to be repaired or replaced in the other, I realized that the stressors I was experiencing in that moment were nothing compared with what this man and dog must face daily. I also felt really good that I hadn't made a big deal about him holding the cup and that I was able to help him and his tiny dog, even just a little bit.

Getting out of our own heads by helping others can give us perspective, which can help reduce our distress level. Things can seem a lot more manageable. And comparing our situation to others is not about sadistically finding joy in someone else's pain. It's actually a worthwhile skill to be able to realize that things could be worse and to be very grateful that they're not.

Real-World Activity:
Step Outside Yourself and Help Others

Which act of kindness will you commit to practicing the next time you feel distress and want to get outside of yourself to skillfully cope?

- help an elderly person with grocery bags?

- pay the adoption fee for a shelter animal?

- offer to do someone else's chore or work task?

- read a book to a young relative?

- call a relative that you know will appreciate the connection?

- surprise someone by thoughtfully picking out a card and mailing it?

- send someone a thank you note?

- pay for the coffee of whoever is standing in line behind you?

- something else?

After you do this random act of kindness, take note of how you feel.

Building Emotional Resiliency

Tolerating distress on a small scale in the ways described here will begin to make a huge difference in your life as you practice doing this over time. These little inoculations will help you build the emotional resiliency you need to handle more substantial life situations as they arise.

Here's another example for you. Having done so much work to overcome the oppressive symptoms of borderline personality disorder, and just when I thought my life was going to be significantly easier to manage, life threw me a major curveball. In March of 2014, I was diagnosed with multiple sclerosis, or MS. Multiple sclerosis is a serious and progressive immune system disease that affects the central nervous system, including the brain and spinal cord. It causes inflammation in these areas, which then damages the myelin sheath covering around nerves that transmit messages to and from the brain and spinal cord to other parts of the body. Because you never know where in the body the next attack will strike, the types and levels of disability experienced from person to person with MS vary. The unpredictability of the disease can serve as an almost constant source of low-level anxiety in the background of life for the sufferer.

If you or someone you love is coping with a chronic illness, you may relate to this topic more than if you have no experience with it. Whatever your situation may be, my hope is that this story shows how working on distress management skills can equip you to handle whatever life-changing events may come your way.

Prior to learning DBT skills, if I had learned that I had this disease (or if I had needed to go through the battery of tests and exams leading up to the diagnosis), I'm sure I would have become so out of balance emotionally that I would have landed in the psychiatric ward. I simply would not have been able to cope. Distress management helped me get through not only the weeks leading up to my diagnosis but also the moment when I heard the news and received this diagnosis. I realize how fortunate I am to have developed these skills before this ordeal began.

My best example of how practicing mindfulness and managing distress can reduce unnecessary suffering happened last winter in the emergency room. For weeks, I had been feeling weak in my legs and complaining of a sense of heaviness in them and in my sacral area. My neurologist was on vacation, and the doctor on call consulted with another neurologist who suggested putting me on oral steroids rather than my usual course of IV therapy during a flare-up. Unfortunately, the oral dosage was not strong enough, and within a week or so, I was unable to walk. I could barely put one foot in front of the other. To move myself forward even a few inches was an incredible struggle, and I had to sit down and rest.

Initially, I panicked and feared the worst: that I was permanently losing the ability to walk and would be wheelchair bound. When I caught myself thinking this way, I was able to call upon my skills to coach myself to be mindful and in the present moment, correcting my catastrophic thought-jumping with statements such as *I am having difficulty walking in this moment. That's all that is happening now, and that's all I can deal with at this time* and *I've had flare-ups with other symptoms that greatly improved with treatment, and this situation can turn out similarly* and *Getting myself worked up right now is only going to further activate my nervous system and make me feel worse all around. I need to work to calm down.*

This is probably a good time to mention that since being diagnosed with MS, I have found that my body now serves me, as an emotionally sensitive person, as a very large barometer of my emotional state. Because our emotions affect our nervous system, and vice versa, I now actually experience and notice physical sensations when I am feeling upset emotionally. Stress, anxiety, and anger, for example, all show up as various levels of transient numbness and tingling in my limbs and other parts of my body. More than one neurologist has informed me of how important stress management is, because activating the nervous system in this way only serves to increase physical symptoms. This is true even if you don't have MS. I am now more aware than ever of when I need to use DBT. This side effect of the disease is actually something I'm using to remind myself to stay as calm and as skillful as possible.

So, after the skillful self-talk to calm myself down, I called a loved one and asked for a ride to the emergency room. Upon arrival, I had to be pushed in a wheelchair to the hospital entrance. I was put on IV steroids and told that they would not discharge me until I showed that I was able to walk. I didn't like this news. It both angered and frightened me. I was afraid to stay in the ER overnight, and that was definitely where it looked like things were heading. I tried to resist and fight the reality of the moment: I couldn't walk, and I was going to be sleeping in the hospital.

It was then that I had the clarity to realize that this was a real-life major opportunity to practice distress tolerance skills. There I was, facing something incredibly uncomfortable and distressing. It was an unwanted situation over which I had zero control. No amount of problem solving in the world would change the circumstances of that moment. And yet I had a choice. I was at a fork in the road, at which I could have engaged in nonproductive, resisting, suffering-causing behaviors, or I could choose the DBT path, using my skills to effectively tolerate the distress of not being able to walk and of needing to stay in the ER for at least twenty-four hours.

I chose the latter, and my experience completely shifted. I was genuinely super kind and engaging with all the medical professionals who visited my room. I paid attention when they spoke and calmly asked them questions about my concerns. I complied with the medical tests and procedures that I needed to undergo. I was no longer fighting reality. I decided to turn on the television. I watched a few sitcoms and allowed myself to use these as a distraction. Even though watching the shows and having a few laughs didn't change my situation, it did pull my attention somewhere else, distracting my thoughts for a little bit, which helped.

That evening, I chose to use acceptance around the fact that I needed to be pushed in a wheelchair multiple times to and from the bathroom. Rather than plunge into full-on crying spells (and believe me, the urge was there), I noticed the emotional reaction I was having and then reminded myself, each time, that I was going to the restroom in the wheelchair *this* time. It didn't mean I would need to be in one the next time or forevermore. I didn't know what the future held, and in that moment, it didn't matter. I only needed to cope with that moment. I inwardly expressed gratitude that I was fortunate enough to have medical insurance and to live in a place with access to good treatment. I outwardly expressed my gratitude to the medical staff who were assisting me. When I noticed fear-inducing thoughts creeping up that didn't serve me in the moment, I imagined putting them in that box up on the shelf to be dealt with, one at a time, at the appropriate moment, and as needed. This all helped substantially.

Through life's challenges, we can grow so much. If we reflect on how our challenges have helped shape and strengthen us, as well as how these situations inevitably produce opportunities to practice being skillful and reduce our suffering, we will be changed by every experience. These experiences can cause us to grow in empathy, which in turn helps us deepen our relationships with others. Life is full of painful events and experiences, but suffering is optional. It is only through situations that have the potential for suffering, and that perhaps at least initially cause us to have some suffering, that we can connect with the truth of this statement for ourselves. Oh, and by the way, my walking was fully restored a few months after this incident!

Real-World Activity:
Note Difficult Events That Brought
Meaning to Your Life

Think about some things that have occurred in your life that at the time felt immensely difficult and perhaps even insurmountable. Recall how your inner strength and resiliency allowed you to ride out these storms. Celebrate that the situation, no matter how difficult or upsetting, had some silver lining that created meaning, and write about this in your notebook.

As you looked back on these periods of your life, were you able to identify at least one or more ways in which some aspect of the situation went on to be meaningful in your personal journey? Perhaps you were stretched further than you thought possible but still bounced back. Perhaps you learned more about who you really are or whom you can really count on. Perhaps you survived something tragic and now have the insight and empathy to help countless others in similar situations to not lose hope.

Keep Choosing Skills over Sabotage

Keep in mind as you continue moving forward and learning new skills that when upset strikes and you find yourself in distress, old habits die hard. The temptation will always be there for us to take the easy, familiar route of old, unskillful behaviors because we've grown so used to using them. We must remind ourselves that these behaviors make us feel better only momentarily and have consequences for our short- and long-term goals, and that's no longer acceptable to us. We're learning new skills, becoming more accountable, and building the life that we want to live. When you catch yourself thinking *I can't handle this*, notice the thought and then change it to *I am handling this*, and begin practicing your distress management skills.

Chapter 3

Regulating Your Emotions

The next step in learning how to better tolerate distress is to look at what you can do to support your overall sense of emotional balance and wellness. This chapter offers some concepts and skills that will help you regulate your emotional reactivity, decreasing your vulnerability and increasing your resiliency. I'll start with a story about how DBT has helped me regulate my emotional reactions and then introduce some exercises that have worked for me and many others.

Dealing with Emotional Reactivity

Before receiving treatment, my emotional reactions, specifically the intensity with which I experienced them and my inability to modulate them, caused me a world of suffering. The other day, I had an opportunity to reflect on how far I have come, as I was sitting in the dentist's chair getting some extensive work done. For nearly a decade, I avoided going to the dentist like the plague. I was so afraid! My oral hygiene suffered, of course, and it wasn't until I was at the point that I needed a root canal and understood the seriousness of my situation that I made a concerted effort to rectify my avoidance.

Through problem solving, I found a very kind, patient, gentle dentist who worked with me and my anxiety. We worked together on an effective technique called *exposure*. The idea with this practice is that you make it a goal, in small increments, to expose yourself to whatever you fear until you can handle it with ease. People who suffer from phobias use this technique to ride in an elevator or fly on an airplane or to get over their fear of dogs. In my case, I needed to keep going to the dentist, over and over and over again, until my fear decreased and the anxiety no longer had a grip on me. I needed lots of appointments to get several dental issues worked out, and each time that I pushed myself to go and take care of myself, my confidence grew in my ability to handle going to the dentist. With each appointment, my anxiety decreased, I lost less sleep the night before, and the panic symptoms were a little less when I got into the dental office. I became more and more at ease being there. Fast-forward a couple of years later to this appointment I had the other day, and I actually was looking forward to going to the dentist! I'm not kidding. Now, you might think this is the opposite extreme, but here's what happened for me.

I faced my fears by showing up, over and over again. I allowed myself to be okay with the fact that I was afraid, as I reassured myself that I was in competent hands and that following through would allow me to take better care of my health. I allowed my body to go through the process of anxiety symptoms, noticing nervous jitters, my racing heart, and clammy hands, while carefully slowing down my breathing so that the symptoms didn't escalate. I began to socialize more with the office staff. I enjoyed interacting with them. And, after getting through what I consider the worst part of what is required at some dental appointments, the injection of Novocain to numb the area, I found it was smooth sailing! Now I just lie back, pop in my earbuds, and relax while listening to soothing jazz from my smartphone.

Because I've worked so hard to manage the emotional intensity of needing to go to the dentist, I no longer get so anxious that I cancel my appointments or lose sleep the night before or have much anxiety prior to dental appointments, and I no longer have panic or anxiety attacks during my visits. But, just when you think you've mastered something, life can cleverly throw a new challenge into the mix. Such was the case at my latest appointment. I showed up confidently, got in the chair, received a shot of Novocain, and was ready to pop in my earbuds when suddenly my heart began to race and my hands began to tremble uncontrollably. I was seriously confused. I called out for my dentist and explained that I didn't know why I was anxious. In fact, I didn't feel anxious or scared at all, yet my heart was racing and my hands were shaking. She informed me that she didn't think it actually was anxiety. I was having a reaction to the epinephrine in the medication, something that had never happened before. I'm not going to lie. I got a bit scared. That began to induce some actual anxiety, and I decided to act fast in getting skillful to get ahold of my mind, body, and emotions.

I knew that if I didn't take things down a notch and begin to soothe and calm my nervous system, I would end up feeling so much worse, both physically and mentally. My dentist rather intuitively began to use helpful language, telling me that my experience was "perfectly normal," that "this happens sometimes," and that the experience would be "transient." Her reassuring words helped normalize the situation and helped me stay grounded in the here and now: *My heart is racing in this moment. It doesn't mean it's going to get worse. It's transient and will subside.*

It can be very helpful to focus on external reassurances when they are being offered, especially in a particular moment when our emotional intensity interferes with our ability to reassure ourselves. When we are feeling heightened emotionally, it can be very easy to overlook or underplay the helpful cues in our environment and to be receptive and responsive only to those cues that will fuel the heightened emotion further, for example, in this case focusing on fear thoughts such as *Oh my god! Do I need to call 9-1-1?* Before DBT, I probably would have focused on those very thoughts. I would have become so terrified and inconsolable that I would have called for an ambulance right there in the dentist chair. Fortunately, that didn't happen this time.

So, why didn't it happen? How can those of us who are emotionally sensitive keep ourselves from being swept up and carried away into escalating spirals of emotional overwhelm? That's what this chapter is all about. Once we acknowledge that we have a problem with emotion dysregulation and believe that by grasping this fact and learning to better manage our emotional experiences, we can improve our life for the better, we are confronted with the challenge of learning skills that can help us do just that: regulate our emotions.

I didn't end up calling 9-1-1, because I was able to stay grounded, or present, in the situation. I noticed the sensations in my body, and when a scary thought arose, I noticed that it was just a thought. These choices prevented the circumstances from driving me into an even more intense state of anxiety. I stayed reasonable by discussing with my dentist what I was noticing and asking her for feedback on her medical interpretation of what was happening. When she responded, instead of dismissing what she was saying, not paying full attention, and getting caught up in my fears, I listened and took deep breaths. Mind you, I was still nervous about the physiological sensations in my body, but I kept reminding myself that a racing heart and tremors would only get worse if I didn't stay as calm as possible. It worked. Within about ten minutes, my heart rate had returned to normal, my hands weren't shaking, and I hadn't had an emotional meltdown. Success!

Listening to Emotions

Emotions are great communicators. Emotions communicate something about our personal, inner experience to others. If you're grinding your teeth, clenching your fists, and your face is beet red, an observer could safely assume that you're angry. We are hardwired to perceive the emotions of others. This innate ability allows us to empathetically relate, take care of each other, and keep ourselves safe. I know that if I were in a room with someone who looked angry, I might excuse myself or, if safe to do so, attempt to help diffuse the situation. What happens sometimes with those of us who are emotionally sensitive is that we take what we observe about others' emotions to another level by adding on our own story or an interpretation that may or may not be true.

We may automatically believe that the person is not just angry but angry *with us*, even without any observable, objective facts to support this. To keep our suffering to a minimum and our emotional regulation to a maximum in interpersonal situations, it's important that when we observe someone else having an emotional experience, we stick to the facts of what we can observe through our senses, without adding our story or interpretation to it. I'll talk more about the importance of this practice in chapter 4, but suffice to say for now that it's a good idea to get into this habit when it comes to understanding what others are communicating to you through their emotional experience.

What Your Emotions Tell You About Yourself

In addition to communicating to others, our emotions can give us vital information about ourselves. They can give us insight into our experience and lead us toward getting our needs met and taking care of ourselves, if we allow the time and space to acknowledge them. One way to become more aware of your emotions is to spend five minutes of silence doing a mindfulness breathing exercise. This allows thoughts and feelings to bubble to the surface. When you are doing nothing except sitting and breathing, you can to listen to your feelings and respond. Try doing this.

Real-World Activity:
Listen to Your Emotions

Get into a comfortable position in a space where you will not be disturbed for the next five minutes. You may want to set a timer so you won't have to look at your watch or the clock. Then sit quietly and simply breathe in and out, counting to yourself each time you inhale and exhale. Count ten breaths and then repeat. Continue counting your breaths this way until the five minutes has elapsed.

Afterward, write about your experience in your notebook. Was sitting for five minutes in silence hard or easy to do? What did you notice about your experience? What feelings came up? Perhaps you noticed other things, such as your thoughts, physical sensations, and sounds in the environment. Describe what you noticed and observed during your practice.

If you had difficulty noticing or identifying your feelings, the next part of this chapter will be helpful. Also, if you find it hard to sit in quiet for five minutes, go easy on yourself. Take a break. Come back to this exercise when you can. Those five minutes used to be intolerable for me when I first learned how to do this in group practice. I'd try to talk my way out of having to do it. I'd get tight and tense in my body. I'd sometimes disregard the instruction and discreetly engage in some other activity. What I realized was that I had a really difficult time sitting still, in quiet, being observant of my experience, because it scared me. When I would actually do the exercise, I would often have experiences that were intensely emotional. Sitting in a chair in a silent room for five minutes with just me and my thoughts and emotions often led to my breaking down in tears. I'd then feel weak, embarrassed, and sad, because I didn't yet have the insight into why this emotion was showing up in that moment (it finally had a chance to do so!), and it felt really intense, which was uncomfortable. Judging myself harshly as being weak only reinforced and escalated my emotional state.

Nowadays, I look forward to this five-minute practice and the inevitable, familiar pattern of resistance that shows up right before I do it. I know that I won't necessarily cry, and if I do cry, I know that it is not a sign of weakness and is nothing to be embarrassed about. Crying communicates to us that we feel sad, and this is information that we can work with. We can tend to ourselves with compassion, explore more deeply why we feel sad, and be present with that emotion, so we can heal through it. This particular experience still happens to me sometimes. It's usually when I have, in fact, been avoiding facing an upsetting issue. Sometimes to avoid sadness, I have found myself voluntarily drowning in work at the computer for ten hours a day without human contact (other than online)—totally not balanced living and a red flag that I'm avoiding the messages my emotions would communicate if I were to allow myself to slow down and feel them. When I get in these ruts of avoiding my emotions, they inevitably surface anyway, louder than they probably would have if I'd tended to them at the onset. Experiencing an outburst of frustrated crying or feeling a sensation of heaviness or anxiety in the pit of my stomach is like an SOS signal. What is being communicated? It's really time to pay attention! Yes, this means being willing to be vulnerable and to feel some pain, but these difficult emotions are not going to go away unless we allow ourselves to experience and move through them, and the pain will only get worse the longer we put it off.

In addition to grabbing our attention and providing us with important information, emotions serve to prompt us to take some sort of action. For example, after acknowledging my sadness and deciding that I want to reduce it in a skillful way rather than just ignore it, I can work on taking some steps to create more balance in my daily life, such as going to a yoga class to get grounded in my body and to be around other people for a while. I can also commit to bringing up the issue that is causing this sadness, either in my next therapy session or with a trusted loved one, to get the support and encouragement I'm needing.

So, even though emotions, especially intense and uncomfortable ones, get a bad reputation and we are inclined to want to avoid them, each and every emotion that presents itself to us serves a purpose. Each brings an important message. We need to give these messages our attention and work on nurturing ourselves through the emotional experience. This is good self-care.

But what if you can't clearly articulate your emotional experience? I used to describe most of my intense emotional experiences as "overwhelm" or "a jumble" because it didn't seem possible to sort out and separate the number of things I was feeling all at once. I just knew I felt bad. Part of the process of regulating your emotions is to become more familiar with what you are truly feeling, what your emotions are communicating to you, so you can accurately express that experience.

Dissecting Your Emotional Experiences

When it comes to emotional experiences, there is a lot of value in being willing to sit down and dissect, piece by piece, element by element, all of the components involved, because doing so can greatly assist you with your goal of regulating your emotions. This exercise is appropriate to use any time you're dealing with a situation in which it would be helpful to listen to what your emotions are trying to tell you. Here's how.

STEP 1: NAME THE EMOTION

Do you feel sad? Angry? Jealous? Anxious? Sometimes we feel such a hodgepodge of emotions that all we know is that we feel bad or overwhelmed. It really is helpful to look beyond that, though, a bit closer, to define our emotional experience. Doing this helps us get grounded in reality and allows us to try to solve the problem. As you work on naming the emotion, take refuge in knowing that emotional experiences, including the distressing one that prompted you to do this exercise, are shared across humanity, and the things we think and want to do in reaction to our emotions are usually quite common.

We're not alone. There isn't something wrong with us. You want to throw something? Sounds like anger. (You don't have to actually throw something, but the urge to do so is common for many people when they get angry.) Regardless of the emotion, if you name it to your therapist or in a group therapy setting while sharing this exercise, most people will either nod or otherwise express that they've been there, too.

When we know what we're feeling, we can take better care of ourselves, let others know what is going on with us, and take steps to address the emotion at hand. For example, I may be feeling overwhelmed with emotion and discover that at the core of my sense of overwhelm is actually fear. The fear, as I dig deeper, is of being single (alone) forever, because I've been single for a while and have felt really lonely lately. My mind, in the form of automatic fear-fueled thoughts, may jump to distressing catastrophizing thoughts, such as *I'm going to be alone forever*. Rather than believe everything I think, getting swept up in despair and intense emotion at such a terrible thought, I can notice and separate the thought out as a thought instead of a fact (*I am single and alone right now, as are millions of people on this planet. I could meet someone someday. Being alone now doesn't mean I'm doomed to be alone forever. I can be alone right now and be okay*). I can then begin to think of ways to address my loneliness, such as making plans to connect with others, getting out of the house more, and sending some e-mails.

Note that at this point in the exercise, you're not actually trying to solve anything; you're just trying to accurately identify your emotion. If you have some insights into problem solving, you can definitely use them later. If you're still having difficulty identifying or pinpointing the main emotion that you are feeling, you can use a "feelings wheel" (a quick Google search will pull up some good ones), or you can work your way through the rest of the steps in this exercise, gathering clues along the way, which may help you identify what it is you are truly feeling. Either way, discovering the main emotion you're experiencing during emotional dysregulation allows you to mindfully examine your experience and get the most out of this practice.

STEP 2: RATE THE EMOTION'S STRENGTH

Rate the strength of your emotion on a scale of 1 to 10, with 1 being very minimal intensity and 10 being the worst ever, the most intolerable or strongest, emotional experience. Be sure to note this. You'll rate the emotion's strength again at the very end of the exercise to observe whether your efforts at problem solving have had any impact in reducing the emotion's intensity as well as your suffering. This is important information to collect.

STEP 3: WHAT'S BEEN GOING ON?

This is the time to take into consideration any emotional and physical issues going on for you that may be contributing to your current dysregulated emotional state. We're only human, and there are certain things, such as not getting enough sleep, forgetting to eat lunch, having a fight with your significant other before leaving for work, or being triggered last night by a movie with a violent scene, that can cause emotional dysregulation and set us up to be more susceptible to being swept up into other intense emotions later.

Or maybe, like me, you have a chronic illness, and it just hasn't been a good day as far as that goes. Have you been feeling well physically? If you have a headache, a cold, or the flu, you're actually not going to be able to call on the same level of emotional resiliency that you have access to when you're feeling in top physical shape. During these times, your energy needs to be conserved for physical recovery, so you may have less patience or less ability to think things through as clearly as you normally would.

With compassion, take a look at your emotional vulnerability factors. When I do this step, I often find myself realizing things like *No wonder I got so angry when she didn't come to pick me up on time. I barely slept last night, and I'm emotionally vulnerable right now.* Whereas I may have been able to tolerate a friend being a few minutes late to pick me up on another day, I just didn't have the emotional reserves on this one, and it's understandable. That being said, of course, being emotionally vulnerable isn't a free pass for us to act out on our emotions with no regard for others, such as lashing out at said friend upon her arrival. However, identifying the things that set us up to have difficulties in situations involving an intense emotion can give us, and others, valuable information about how the situation got out of hand.

Use this information to show yourself compassion, and if you've acted in a way that you regret, and your actions have affected someone who is a caring, supportive person in your life, you might consider sharing whatever has made it difficult for you to cope in an effective way in this latest situation. Most people understand that we all get overwhelmed sometimes and may lose our cool for a minute. If your loved one graciously forgives you, make it a point to do your very best to be mindful not to go there again with the same type of behavior the next time you're feeling an intense emotion. This can help build trust, and it's going to take effort. Believe me, because I know. It will mean deliberately not letting stressors pile up before addressing them, openly communicating when you're struggling, and taking care of yourself while using skills.

STEP 4: DESCRIBE YOUR THOUGHTS (INCLUDING ASSUMPTIONS, BELIEFS, AND JUDGMENTS)

The idea is to review, as objectively as possible, each thought you are having and consider whether it may be fear based or otherwise so emotionally charged that it may not actually be true. We can save ourselves a whole world of suffering by taking this step.

One of the most complicated things about being human—and that can be amplified if you have BPD, past trauma, or emotional sensitivity—is a tendency to believe that our thoughts are facts, or at least those thoughts that come along with intense emotions (see chapter 1). For example, have you ever made a tiny mistake at work and your brain jumped to this thought: *Oh my gosh. I'm going to lose my job! They are going to fire me!?* Then, in the intensity of that emotional experience, you found yourself in the pit of despair? Maybe you then impulsively quit your job or began to check out emotionally, figuring you're going to lose the job anyway. Chances are, in most situations, a tiny mistake wouldn't be cause for being fired, and yet you were reacting as if the opposite were true. This type of automatic, worst-case scenario thinking is something to really be aware of and to challenge. It's upsetting, and it confuses other people, creating more overall emotional dysregulation.

Here's another example. Have you ever been in a romantic relationship, and during a particular conversation, your significant other seemed disinterested in what you had to say? Did you then leap in your mind from seeing signs of disinterest to *He doesn't love me anymore. He's going to leave me. He's cheating!?* Then, without saying anything about it to your significant other, did you begin behaving in a mean way or begin withdrawing? Perhaps you were convinced that if you had those fearful thoughts, accompanied by such deep emotions as fear, anger, and rejection, it must be true. Imagine the confusion of a romantic partner in those moments. For me, this scenario used to happen all the time!

These are two common examples of believing a thought without checking for supporting facts. Not everything we think is true. As you observe your thought process, you give yourself the opportunity to take a step back and evaluate the truthfulness of each thought to the best of your ability while engaging your rational mind.

STEP 5: NOTICE BODY SIGNALS

Next, notice what you are feeling in your body and what you are expressing through your body language. You might take a few moments to scan yourself from head to toe, noticing the places where sensation is more obvious. Perhaps there is tension present in certain areas. Are you clenching your jaw? Are your shoulders tight? How about your neck muscles? Are you clenching your teeth? Continue down the rest of the body. My students are often surprised to discover back pain, a feeling of tightness somewhere else in the body, and even a headache that they hadn't noticed before. It's amazing what we can discover about what's going on in our bodies when we take a moment to focus on nothing but what's happening inside of us.

The information you gather during this step is also incredibly helpful for understanding the emotion you're experiencing and how you can get cues from your body in the future to help you identify what's going on emotionally. This can be especially useful if you have not yet identified your emotion back in step 1 of this exercise. So how can your body give you cues about what you feel emotionally? As an example, if you're experiencing tightness and clenching in your jaw, tension in your shoulders and neck, and a headache, what emotion do you imagine you might be experiencing? Is it intense anxiety and fear? Perhaps anger? Are you also slouching? Is your head in your hands? Are you clenching your fists? Are you maybe feeling defeated or sad?

Being aware of how your body automatically responds or reacts during an emotional episode can be very revealing. It also empowers you to take action to care for yourself on a physical level, which in turn can help relax your nervous system and bring you mental relief. The physical and mental are interconnected. When I'm experiencing intense anxiety, I almost always have the physical sensations of tension that I just described. At these times, I turn to things like autogenics, which is a relaxation technique where you train your body to respond to suggestions such as *My heart is beating slow and steady. My arms are heavy. My legs are warm.* My therapist told me that this technique works by "going backwards" to relaxation through deliberate thought, entering through the parasympathetic nervous system, where these sensations of heaviness, warmth, and a slow, steady heartbeat would be activated if relaxation were invoked already.

I also like to use Yoga Tune Up balls. You can use these to give yourself a gentle massage and get deeper into some muscles, like the trapezius, a muscle in the upper back near the shoulders that is often very tight and in pain when we're anxious. My yoga teacher shared with me that soothing through touch can have a profound impact on the nervous system, allowing it to disengage from threat (fight-or-flight) mode. You may have other techniques that you like to use or have yet to explore and discover, such as taking a brisk walk, doing yoga, meditating, sculpting, or dancing. Do whatever calms your nervous system to reduce that emotion and your suffering. This step of observing your physical experience allows you to then choose to address it with loads of compassionate self-care; this process can be life changing, allowing you to more readily identify stressful emotions and address them early on before they lead to unwanted behaviors.

STEP 6: NOTICE THE URGES

Inevitably, as you're having intense thoughts and feelings, there will be accompanying urges. If your thinking patterns and feelings are primarily anxious, you may have the urge to run, to hide, or to avoid a situation. If you're angry, you might have the urge to yell, to throw something, or to attack. It's important at this point to distinguish between urges and actions; actions will be addressed in the next step. Urges and actions are different. You can have the most powerful of urges but still choose to not act on them. This may seem next to impossible in a moment of severe emotional dysregulation, but it's the truth. Every urge will eventually pass. Every urge has its natural progression of becoming intense, peaking, and then coming down again. And we have a choice each and every time to respond to the urge or to let it pass.

If you've ever managed to successfully quit smoking (I have!) or quit using any other substance, you can tap into the essence of this truth. That urge for a cigarette can come on like nobody's business. You feel like you must have a cigarette or the whole world will fall apart. You think you might absolutely lose it if you don't have one. Then you distract yourself. You have a piece of gum. You go for a walk. You stay away from sources of cigarettes. You call a friend for support around sticking with your goal. Within a relatively short amount of time, the urge subsides. You made a different, more skillful choice. The urge was to smoke, but because you have health goals that involve reducing or avoiding smoking, you chose a different action. You noticed the urge and let it go.

STEP 7: NOTICE YOUR ACTIONS

This part of the exercise is not about judging yourself. It's more about taking the time to notice what actions you chose to take, evaluating the effectiveness of those actions in furthering your well-being, and then using this information to prepare yourself to cope more effectively the next time you feel triggered to act or behave the same way. Did you get angry with your friend for canceling plans, have the urge to slam down the phone and unfriend her online, but then decide to give yourself a day before responding, so you could keep your cool? Perhaps you felt anxious about going to a party and had the urge to avoid it, so you called and made an excuse and didn't attend.

If you do not like an action that you took, you can use this exercise as a learning opportunity. By taking the time to think this process through, you have created a memory that you can draw upon the next time you notice the same signs and signals (see steps 5 and 6). When you feel the urge to act in a way that has not served you well in the past, you can notice it and then remind yourself that having an urge doesn't mean you have to act on that urge. You can choose to put up a mental stop sign, distract yourself, engage in self-care, put time and space between the urge and any action, and make a new and healthier choice.

STEP 8: NOTICE THE AFTEREFFECTS

An intense bout of anxiety may leave you feeling completely exhausted. After an angry episode, you might feel shame or remorse. Notice how you feel emotionally and physically after the intense emotional experience you've been dissecting. This is about being aware of the full picture. It's about understanding the aftereffects we experience in our minds and bodies as a result of our emotions and our responses and reactions to them. There are consequences. As time goes on and you repeat this exercise in different situations, notice whether the aftereffects of your experience begin to change in any way. I've definitely noticed that if I choose a skillful action in response to an urge and then engage in loads of self-care and quiet time, the aftereffects are much less intense than they would have been otherwise. This encourages me to make skillful choices again the next time around.

Remember that you won't be perfect at this. It's hard to believe how many times I've found myself in the same place again, having a full-on panic attack and getting to the point of exhaustion shortly thereafter. Remember too that our bodies have ingrained physiological responses to emotions. We can do our best to soothe our nervous system and to use the skills we are learning, but there will be times when we can continue to feel unwell. If I have used my skills and still feel distressed with anxiety, I may use a medication prescribed by my psychiatrist. I may call my therapist. It is important to be flexible and be willing to do what it takes to help yourself return to emotional equilibrium, especially when you've been severely dysregulated. It's okay to reach out to your treatment team, doctor, therapist, or other support person. You do not need to go through the aftereffects alone.

STEP 9: RATE THE EMOTION'S STRENGTH AGAIN

Rating the emotion's strength at the end of this exercise can be a really positive reinforcement when the intensity has decreased. It tells you that something worked, and you then get to evaluate the worth of the exercise for future use. If the emotion stayed steady or did not decrease in intensity, try to figure out why. Did you act on the urge instead of allowing it to pass so that you could make a more skillful choice? Does the threat that incited the emotion still exist? If you are seeing a therapist, be sure to check in about this experience and ask for suggestions and insights on what shifts might allow for a reduction of intensity in the future.

Dissect Your Emotional Experience

The next time you have an intense emotion, give this exercise a try. Keep a record in your notebook. Here, again, are the steps:

1. Name the emotion.

2. Rate the emotion's strength.

3. What's been going on?

4. Describe your thoughts (including assumptions, beliefs, and judgments).

5. Notice body signals.

6. Notice the urges.

7. Notice your actions.

8. Notice the aftereffects.

9. Rate the emotion's strength again.

How are you feeling now? Has the urge to act in a destructive way gone down? Usually by the time I finish with this type of exercise, the urge to act in a destructive way has decreased so much that I no longer feel compelled to act on it.

With time and practice, you may get to the point where noticing and evaluating your experience begins to come more intuitively and automatically, and this, of course, will happen as a result of practice and commitment to these skills.

Getting Out of the Rut

Okay, you've been in the lab a few times now. You've done some hard work and have been taking the time to really look at your experiences and reflect on your emotions and behaviors. It's time to take a break. There needs to be a balance. You do not need to constantly be in self-fix-it mode. This can lead to burnout and emotional dysregulation. On the other hand, while it may feel like the natural thing to sit around in sweatpants isolating and ruminating when you're not feeling well emotionally, that type of response, at least in excess, can actually be very counterproductive to feeling regulated emotionally.

Doing things to improve your mood, even in small baby steps and little doses, allows you to gather up positive, affirmative experiences. These experiences help you feel better in the moment while you're doing them, and they can have lasting effects. You feel good, and as a result, you feel motivated and encouraged to seek out more of these experiences. And please don't confuse self-care with self-indulgence. So many of us emotionally sensitive people have long believed the lie that we deserve to be punished and to feel miserable, and we often inflict that punishment on ourselves, sometimes by withholding opportunities for positive experiences. Through skillfulness, with the goal of emotional regulation in mind, we can move away from this mentality and begin to make healthier decisions.

So, get out of the house and go have that decaf soy mocha at your favorite cafe and be around other humanoids. Go see that matinee on a weekday. Call up a friend you haven't seen in a while and have a nice meal together. Take a drive up the coast. Start reading that new book you've heard so much about. Take that bubble bath. Go for a walk in that quaint town a few miles away. Do things that make you feel good. It's okay! At first it may feel weird or awkward or unnatural or as if you *should be doing something else more productive*. I know that when I first started practicing this skill, it felt awkward. I felt guilty, like I didn't do anything to deserve feeling good.

However, I came to consider this type of thought as an *old tape*. I learned to simply notice those old tape thoughts, call them out for what they were (untrue messages I came to believe about my supposed lack of worthiness), and follow through on my positive activities. Doing this works! Please be kind to yourself. Notice those old tapes when they come up and then gently silence them. You're writing a new song now. You're the author. You're making healthier choices and taking better care of yourself. You know it's in your best interest to treat yourself with kindness and to allow yourself opportunities to enjoy life. That's what you deserve.

Turning That Frown Upside Down

Another self-regulation skill is to do the opposite of your emotional urge. This is not the same as suggesting that nothing is wrong. You can do the opposite of your emotional urge while recognizing that underneath you are still struggling with some type of difficulty and that there's a pain that is seeking to be acknowledged, processed, and healed. This suggestion is to actually engage in some practical behaviors that will help.

To do this effectively, it's important to remember that every emotion has an urge to act a certain way associated with it. When we're angry, we typically have the urge to lash out or attack. When we're scared or anxious, we typically have the urge to hide. When we're sad, the urge is usually to retreat, isolate, and curl up and become small. If you are experiencing an emotion that is no longer serving you or is out of proportion to the event that prompted it, and you want to reduce your suffering, instead of engaging in the urge that comes up, you can choose to act the opposite.

So if you're feeling angry at someone, have allowed yourself to acknowledge your anger, and don't want to make matters worse by continuing to express how you feel, you might choose to deliberately shift to a calmer, kinder manner of speaking, even though your blood is still boiling and your hands are still shaking. Likewise, if you're feeling scared or anxious but realize that there's no real threat to your well-being or safety, you might gently approach what you fear rather than avoid it. As an example, maybe there's a social gathering at your new school, and you really want to make some friends, so you decide to go to the gathering rather than stay in your dorm room. Or if it's a rainy day out and you're feeling sad, you might put on your raincoat and head out to class or work instead of staying under the covers all day.

If we act in accordance with an emotion's urge, it only serves to reinforce and fuel it, and we'll continue to feel that emotion, perhaps even more intensely. Again, we always have a choice about whether or how we act on a given urge, no matter how intense it may be. It's actually quite an incredible and powerful experience, when appropriate, to choose to behave in the opposite manner. It takes a lot of willingness to make it happen, because the urge associated with the emotion is the one that is going to take the least amount of energy and thought to act on.

To act in the opposite way takes skillfulness and willingness in the form of slowing down, thinking things through, and making a deliberate choice to go against the grain of what may be a very strong urge. The good news is, if your goal is to regulate your emotions, this skill can be incredibly effective, and like the rest of the skills you're learning, the more you do it, the easier it becomes. Acting opposite to the emotional urge sends an important message to the brain. It interrupts the usual pattern of behavior associated with the upsetting emotion, and it helps us shift gears to the emotion we *want* to experience.

I remember realizing how wonderfully empowering it is to be able to choose to change the course of my emotions. Before learning about DBT, I had no concept of this. I had a lot of knee jerk reactions to my thoughts and emotions, and I felt like I couldn't help my behavior. I even said that to people, "But I can't help it. I just get so upset, and I just instantly …" I thought that my upsetting thoughts and uncomfortable feelings were in charge of me, causing me to act in certain ways. But there absolutely is a moment of choice where we do decide how we'll behave. We may have an intense emotion and an upsetting thought and then feel an urge to do something. No matter how strong the urge, we still have the power to make a decision in that next moment of how we will respond. You now have a new tool in your toolbox to explore when this moment of choice arises.

Real-World Activity:

Change Your Emotion Through Acting Opposite

The next time you have an upsetting emotion that you would like to shift, take out your notebook and try answering the following:

1. Name the emotion.

2. Rate the emotion's intensity on a scale of 1 to 10, where 1 is minimal intensity and 10 is the greatest intensity.

3. What is the urge, or what is the emotion prompting you to do? Will acting on the urge be beneficial to you? Will it help you meet your short- and long-term goals? Will it be helpful in your relationships with others?

4. If acting on the urge will be beneficial in certain ways, you may not need to act the opposite way, but if you still would like to reduce and shift your current emotion, or if acting on the urge will not be beneficial, continue on.

5. What at this time are some examples of how you could act opposite to what the emotion is urging you to do?

6. Are you willing to engage in any of these actions? If so, which one(s)?

7. Before engaging in these new actions, try to validate your emotion. Find the morsel of truth that substantiates why you are feeling this way. For example, *Of course I'm feeling angry. I was insulted.*

8. After choosing to act opposite of your emotional urge, how do you feel?

9. Rate the emotion's intensity again on a scale of 1 to 10, where 1 is minimal intensity and 10 is the greatest intensity.

Your emotion has likely shifted by now. For example, you may have started out feeling fearful but are now feeling content. You may have started out feeling angry but are now feeling much calmer. Did doing the exercise help decrease the emotional intensity? If not, what might have stood in the way?

You can use this exercise of acting opposite anytime you have an upsetting emotion that you would like to shift away from.

Using Visualization

There is one more skill that you can use to help build your confidence and ability to handle situations that you believe will be difficult to navigate emotionally. In relationships, such potentially dysregulating situations can range from knowing you'll have to deal with an annoying coworker when you get to work to having to say good-bye to a loved one who is about to leave on a business trip when you hate being alone. Other potentially dysregulating situations can be mostly about your own inner experience, such as needing to go to an anxiety-provoking medical appointment or having to take an important test. In either case, using visualization to vividly imagine yourself succeeding in the situation can be highly effective. That's why this tool is so popular among professional athletes and other performers.

I have used this skill many times to prepare for certain physical exams, and I know from experience that it works. Practicing planning ahead through visualization not only reduces my anxiety but also helps get me through the appointment itself with far less emotional suffering than I would otherwise experience. You can use this skill to accomplish tasks you need to do for your highest good and best interest when the thought of doing them may provoke intense fear.

Perhaps you have something coming up for which you can apply this skill. To prepare yourself, you would write out a detailed narrative for how you would like things to go, and then you would read and reread the narrative to live out the screenplay in your mind. In doing this, you are training your mind to cope with the actual situation. Here's an example of a visualization in preparation for taking a test at school.

I've just finished breakfast and brushed my teeth. I'm now sitting on the couch, dressed and ready to go, except for my shoes. I've got one hand on my chest and the other on my abdomen. I'm practicing breathing slowly and evenly to support my nervous system in staying calm. I'm inhaling slowly. I'm exhaling slowly. I'm now taking my attention off of my breath and allowing it to return to normal on its own. I'm getting up from the couch. I'm walking toward the shoe rack by the front door. I'm bending down to put on my left shoe. I'm now bending down to put on my right shoe. I'm standing up slowly. I'm reaching for my purse. I'm grabbing my keys from my purse. I'm turning the doorknob to open the door. I'm opening the door. I'm stepping outside. I'm turning the bottom lock on the doorknob. I'm closing the door behind me. I'm locking the top lock with my key. I'm walking down the driveway, one step at a time. I've arrived at my car. Now I'm in my car, settling in comfortably, and now I'm putting the keys in the ignition. I'm turning on the radio to get to my favorite station. Now I'm listening to some soothing jazz as I back down the driveway. I head toward Main Street, stopping at the light and adjusting my rearview mirror. Now I'm passing the church and grocery store, heading to the other end of town. Now I'm at the school. I am pulling into a convenient parking spot. I'm approaching the building, step by step. I'm entering the building and heading to the testing room. I'm walking in, grabbing my test paper, and sitting down. I'm taking a couple of deep breaths, siting up with a confident posture, and I'm now taking the test. I've got this.

While the specifics will vary depending on the situation you are facing, the basic steps are the same for any visualization. You will want to add as much realistic detail as possible as you prepare yourself for handling the situation successfully. After you finish writing the narrative, you read and reread it in preparation for the actual event. The goal is to convince your brain that you are on some level actually having the experience. Adding in as much detail as possible helps accomplish this.

Real-World Activity:
Write (and Live Out) the Screenplay in Your Mind

Do this exercise the next time you want to build your confidence for handling a potentially dysregulating situation. As vividly as possible, in first-person, write out a detailed narrative of how you want the situation to unfold. Imagine yourself successfully navigating the many nuances of the experience, completing it, and moving on with your life. Note every little step along the way, and then read this narrative to yourself over and over until the day of the event. This will help you prepare yourself to cope as best as you possibly can.

The human imagination is incredibly powerful, and many of us who are emotionally sensitive have very vivid imaginations. We often unfortunately use this power to engage in worst-case scenarios and to freak ourselves out with *what-if* catastrophizing, but this exercise gives us yet another opportunity to make a different, healthier, more skillful choice.

Emotionally Healthy People Make Better Friends, Partners, Parents, Employees

Emotional experiences can feel like a triathlon, so we may as well harness the power of visualization in our lives. We can use it to prepare ourselves to behave and cope skillfully when we anticipate a difficult conversation with another person, whether our goal is to preserve our self-respect, get a need met, keep the relationship, or a combination of these. In fact, when it comes to relationships, when we are feeling better, taking good care of ourselves, and better managing our emotions, we are happier and better able to connect with others in healthy, meaningful, and lasting ways.

You now have some ideas about how to notice behaviors or situations that may be impacting your emotional equilibrium and some new tools to help you regulate your emotions and stay strong in the face of distress. The next chapter will dive into taking all of this hard work to the next level: being skillful in relationships.

Chapter 4

Working on Relationships

Okay. Now I'm getting really excited, and I hope you are, too. Ultimately, we learn DBT skills because we want to change our lives for the better. We realize that we have some serious, challenging, and at times uncomfortable work to do, and as the resilient creatures that we have come to be, we set out to do it. We want to reduce our suffering and to enjoy life with less drama and more peace. But is there more to it than that? Sure, we want to feel good in our own skin. We want to feel skillful and to act from a place of integrity. We want to feel healthy and balanced. These aspirations are definitely worth the effort and are incredibly motivating, but something else also strongly motivates us. Underneath it all, at the core, we anticipate what life will look like on a day-to-day basis once we get ourselves "right" and healthy. At the core of it all, we picture ourselves having strong relationships that last. Finally.

As social creatures, we naturally long to truly and deeply connect with others. We want to have (and keep!) meaningful, healthy relationships with people we love and who genuinely, unconditionally, love us right back in equal doses. Yet, without tools to manage intense emotional dysregulation, our success rate has likely been very low up until now. Relationships instead tend to start off wonderfully, become super intense, and then end catastrophically. It becomes tiring and discouraging when, each time you think that this will be the friendship, romantic partnership, or job that will last, another crisis comes to town and the whole thing is sabotaged. The bottom line is that we must make different choices for different outcomes. To do this, we must foster an awareness of these different choices to which, up until now, we haven't had access. DBT skills can help bridge that gap.

Mind Over Mood

Just to keep things real, there are going to be days when you are feeling more emotionally vulnerable than others. At these times, even with the best of intentions and a plan in place to use your skills, a mood swing can really test your resolve. You will need to focus on your skills even more in these moments, so you can handle these situations effectively.

Mood swings are going to happen. There will be times when you will feel like treating your significant other poorly because you're in a bad mood, or you're going to have the urge to withdraw and not follow through on an important commitment, because you "don't feel like it." If you don't know how to handle distress, manage your intense emotions, and be in the present moment, it is, honestly, nearly impossible to have the types of relationships you may romanticize in your mind and seek. You have to continue to work on and fine-tune these interpersonal skills, and these scenarios are just the right opportunities to practice them.

Being in relationships is hard work. I'm not going to pretend that I have mastered the art of being skillful in relationships or that I don't still make unskillful interpersonal blunders. It's also incredibly unlikely that by simply reading this book, you are going to feel and be ready to enter into the world of relationships as a complete and whole person, with no baggage and with a total newfound sense of being able to skillfully and successfully maintain healthy relationships.

It's going to take lots more practicing of skills, taking risks, and being vulnerable, though this time in healthy, not impulsive, ways and not at the cost of your self-respect or your goals or as a result of succumbing to fears of abandonment and rejection. If you are also dealing with past wounds, it will take a lot of work to turn off those old tapes—those pain-skewed, untrue messages you perhaps heard growing up and have grown to believe about yourself and what relationships should be like—that negatively influence your relationships today.

Even so, this chapter will equip you with some powerful, basic interpersonal skills. And the good news is, you're already off to a great start! You've been learning important skills and opening your mind to new options and choices. You're demonstrating a willingness to work on yourself. This is admirable, and your efforts can lead to the most rewarding and fulfilling application of all of this knowledge: the ability to apply it in meaningful ways to build, keep, and repair relationships.

Transformative results don't happen overnight, and again, it's going to take work! Most of us have had a difficult time building, keeping, and repairing our most important relationships. Beyond that, we've even had difficulties interacting effectively with people in everyday situations, such as with a clerk at a store, with another driver on the road, or with a teacher or a boss, because our emotions have gotten the better of us. All of these scenarios can benefit from understanding and using DBT, and a good place to start is to get clear on your interpersonal goals.

Three Main Relationship Goals

It's helpful to look at your relationships in terms of three main goals: getting your needs met assertively, maintaining relationships, and preserving your self-respect. When it comes to choosing and using interpersonal skills, the first step is to identify what your goal is in a particular situation, given the type of relationship(s) involved and the outcome you hope to achieve. At any given time and from one situation to the next, you will begin to prioritize your goals. Then, as you're considering your next steps, the question you'll want to ask is *What choices or actions will likely get me closer to meeting my objective in this situation?*

For example, let's imagine that you have, for the most part, what you consider to be a great job at a clothing design firm. You can hardly believe that with your spotty work history, this company has actually given you a chance. You charmed them and got your foot in the door. Somehow your references checked out. Or maybe they weren't checked. Anyhow, you work alongside creative, fun, and interesting people all day long and love learning all you can, as you secretly aspire to launch your own clothing line at some point. The problem is, despite everything that's going right at this job, you don't care for your boss. At all. And that's putting it lightly.

You find him to be condescending, rude, and, if you're honest, quite incompetent. You dread phone calls from him ("reject call" button, anyone?) and those uncomfortable, massively anxiety-provoking in-person meetings. He doesn't listen to your suggestions and dismisses them in patronizing ways. At times, you're tempted to quit and throw away this opportunity because of how bad you feel around him, even though you manage to stay out of his presence for most of the week. Somehow, you've kept it together so far, but you have begun calling in sick on days when the two of you are scheduled to meet. One of your personal goals is to behave with integrity by being honest and moral in your dealings with others, and you feel completely the opposite of this when you call in sick.

Clearly, you have a dilemma on your hands. Let's look at the interpersonal goals you can choose as your focus. In this situation, you might feel a strong competition between all three relationship goals: wanting to assertively ask for your suggestions to be fairly considered, wanting to maintain the relationship so that you can keep your job, and wanting to preserve your self-respect by communicating that you believe you deserve better treatment. You acknowledge to yourself that you need your job and that your boss has power over whether you continue working there or not. If you decide that the goal of preserving your self-respect, coupled with your desire to assertively get your needs met, wins out, and you're willing to risk the possible consequences associated with taking actions to meet this goal (including losing your job because your boss isn't impressed with your approach), what might be your next move? Perhaps you end up deciding to respectfully and assertively confront your boss about your concerns. You decide to share with him how his demeanor seems condescending, let him know that this is uncomfortable for you, and ask him to speak to you more respectfully.

Now, if preserving your self-respect in this manner could possibly lead to losing your job, and this is just not an option for you at this time (or the mere thought of speaking to your superior in this way already has you in a full-on panic attack), clearly, this isn't the right goal for the situation. If, on the other hand, maintaining the relationship and your job sound like more appealing goals, your course of action is going to look very different. In this case, you'd be evaluating which skills you can use to cope effectively with the upset you feel when your boss is disrespectful, so you don't lose your cool. You'd focus on skills to help you cope effectively with the anxiety that comes up before your meetings, so you no longer avoid them, because repeatedly calling in sick could cause you to lose your job and not accomplish your desired objective. Make sense?

Real-World Activity:
Setting Goals and Objectives

Give it a try for yourself. Here are the steps.

1. Think of an interpersonal situation that is troubling you. Describe it in your notebook. Who is involved, and what is at stake?

2. Rate the importance of your three main interpersonal goals in this situation: getting your needs met assertively, maintaining the relationship, and preserving your self-respect. If it helps, you can rate each goal on a scale of 0 to 10, where 0 means not important at all and 10 means most important.

3. With your main goal in mind, ask yourself what types of behaviors or actions you could take to try to get you closer to your desired objective in this situation. Write down some possible outcomes, including undesired as well as desired outcomes.

Once you have a plan that makes the most sense for you and your objectives, you may want to check in with someone whom you trust before proceeding with it. As you practice this process more and more, you'll become more confident about making this decision for yourself.

Choosing and acting on your interpersonal goals will help you accomplish them. It's also important to keep in mind that sometimes, no matter how skillful you are, you may not accomplish what you set out to achieve. Interactions and relationships are complicated. If others' goals are not in alignment with yours, if they have a different agenda entirely, or if they are unwilling to compromise, your objectives may not be met. If this happens, you must then use skills to cope effectively with disappointment, so you don't react out of anger, revenge, or temporary hopeless feelings or thoughts. Remember, you don't want to make matters worse.

The Benefits of Slowing Things Down

Maybe you've just tried the exercise above and are finding yourself where I once was. You're realizing that there are, indeed, almost always more options than typically meet the eye when you're emotionally dysregulated in your relationships and faced with choosing what to do next. Prior to DBT, I certainly didn't think things through at this level of detail, looking at what I wanted to come out of a situation, what I would need to do to potentially achieve this, what the various outcomes might be, and how I would cope skillfully if I didn't get what I wanted.

I didn't stop to think about how I wanted to feel or what I wanted the situation to look like *after* the interaction. Instead, my raw emotions ran the show. I was impulsive and wanted to feel better *now* and often wanted to experience a sense of satisfaction and self-righteousness in that moment, without giving much thought to the short- and long-term consequences. So, taking the previous example of life in the workplace, like many people with BPD, I have had a lot of jobs. In retrospect, to be effective, what I really needed to do was to slow down and think things through, but I had no such tools for accomplishing this until DBT. Some of the mindfulness skills covered earlier in this book, such as accepting reality, noticing judgments, and doing what works in the situation, can all be very helpful with slowing things down. You can then focus on meeting your desired objective rather than getting swept up into intense emotions that are demanding instant satisfaction and relief.

These DBT skills have helped me slow things down and live more consciously, and they can do the same for you. By taking the time to look at your goals in any situation that involves another person, you give yourself the opportunity to be skillful. You give yourself the opportunity to stop burning bridges. You can stop the unhealthy pattern of destroying connections, jobs, and relationships.

Focusing on Your Interpersonal Goals

Let's take a look at another example of how focusing on an interpersonal goal can help in relationships. Say that you have set the intention to work on the goal of getting your needs met assertively in relationships. Perhaps you find yourself constantly saying yes to someone's requests for your time, even when you are overwhelmed with your own to-do list. Or perhaps it's difficult for you to ask the other person to do something to help you.

Imagine you live with a roommate who is not doing her fair share of the housework. If your main interpersonal goal is get her to pitch in at an equal level, it's going to take you skillfully and tactfully asking in a way that will likely get her to consider your point of view and begin to cooperate. This means being assertive, acknowledging any concerns or objections she may have, and then setting and enforcing your expectations or limits. On the other hand, you may have other interpersonal goals that are more important here than getting your needs met assertively. In situations like this, it may be helpful to slow things down and examine your goals in more detail.

Real-World Activity:
Examining Your Goals

Think of an interpersonal situation you are facing at this time in which you are not getting your needs met. In your notebook, describe the situation in detail, who is involved, what you hope to see happen, and what is at stake if things don't go the way you would like.

Example: *My roommate has stopped doing her fair share of housework. I'm tired of it, as I also work full time and don't think it's fair that I come home and then clean up after her as well. I'd like to see her begin to pitch in equally. If she doesn't agree to do this, I'm not sure I can go on being her roommate.*

Describe what you're thinking and feeling.

Example: *It's actually concerning to me that she suddenly stopped pitching in. I do feel disrespected, which makes me feel angry, but I have a hard time believing that it's her intention to make me feel this way. I'm confused. This isn't like her. We've been roommates for nine months now, and we've been getting along pretty well. I enjoy living with her. She's quiet, pays her share of the rent and bills on time, and we like a lot of the same TV shows. She's a good person. She's been there for me on those eating-a-pint-of-almond-milk-ice-cream breakup nights. I have to wonder if something is going on with her. I don't want to be hasty and jump on her case and get upset. I've lost so many friends that way. I like her, and I can't afford to lose her financial contributions to the household expenses right now. I don't want to be a doormat, but I also don't want to push her away. I don't want be too aggressive.*

This is a lot to consider and balance! On the one hand, I feel disrespected and angry, but I also know that it's unlikely that my roommate intends for me to feel this way—it's not like her. I've enjoyed our friendship for some time now. And while I want to keep my self-respect intact, I'm aware that I also don't want to come off as too aggressive and push her away. I'm angry enough to consider not being roommates with her anymore, but it's also not in my best interest financially to go in that direction at this time. I'm faced with a choice. While my knee-jerk reaction may be to put all of her stuff out on the lawn in an angry rage, some part of me fully knows that this is not going to be in my best interest or in the interest of the relationship.

Next, write down which of your three main interpersonal goals is a priority at this time.

Example: *I will make maintaining the relationship my primary goal in this situation, because we have a history of working things through, being friends, she's a good roommate in general (the TV, paying on time), and I can't afford to make a decision out of anger that will leave me with one less friend and all the bills to handle myself. I can reflect upon and honor the fact that I want to keep my self-respect and be assertive, so I don't feel like a doormat—these are important things, too—but, all things considered, I'll keep my focus on my main goal of maintaining my relationship with my roommate.*

Now think of the behaviors you can engage in that are in alignment with your goal. Describe them in your notebook.

Example: *I'll bring it up gently and ask her what's going on and how she's feeling. Then I'll let her know that I've noticed some of her chores haven't been getting done. Nothing accusatory. Just curiosity. We'll take it from there. We've been able to talk out other things in the past, so there is hope that this can be worked out, too.*

Share your work on this exercise with someone you trust to get some support around skillfully attempting to achieve your goal. Then take actions that are in alignment with your goals and journal about how things went.

Note the words "attempting to achieve your goal." You now have a tool to help you prioritize your interpersonal goals, allowing you to plan how to convey your needs skillfully. However, even with this new skill and all the hard work it will take to practice it, sometimes things still won't go as you'd hoped, and you will have to deal with disappointment.

When Things Don't Go as Planned

Maybe your roommate will still decide to move out even though you tried so hard to ensure that she wouldn't. You thought you did all the right things. When situations don't go as hoped or expected when we're trying a new, more skillful approach, it can be incredibly discouraging and disappointing. However, this can be yet another excellent opportunity to practice skills, because life will have its share of disappointments. Relationships are incredibly complex (and often complicated!), and there are so many different ways an interpersonal scenario can play out.

Sometimes we won't get our way or the other person will respond in an unskillful fashion. Some people may even be suspicious of your efforts to approach things differently from how you have up until now. Handling these scenarios without becoming further dysregulated can be challenging, and it's an important topic, so let's talk about what the world really looks like as you're growing and evolving, telling your friends and relatives about your epiphanies and self-discoveries, and attempting to make new choices that will likely surprise them.

Getting the Validation You Need

As loved ones begin to witness you handling things differently from how you have in the past, as you're making new choices that lead to new outcomes, you'd probably imagine that everyone would be on board and supportive, believing in your ability to succeed and cheering you on. Some will. Others won't, and it's important to be prepared for that. The disappointment and feelings of rejection that come up in these cases will need to be met with skillfulness. Just as there have been people in your life who've had a difficult time affirming and accepting you as an emotionally sensitive person or a BPD sufferer, there will be some people who find it challenging to support your efforts to move your life in a new direction. Some of this might be attributed to their hesitancy to trust that this time you're really changing. Maybe they're afraid of being burned again. That's reasonable, right? Doesn't make it hurt any less, but you can understand their concern.

Other times, people who are close to you can end up actually being emotionally rattled by your changes. Their equilibrium gets disrupted. They are inevitably being pushed to move out of their comfort zone as you change and the nature of your relationship with them is changing. Just as the dynamics in families radically changes when a longtime alcoholic family member becomes sober—codependents in the caretaker role may lose a sense of their identity and purpose and may no longer know how to relate to the sober person—others around you will need to shift and grow as a result of you becoming healthier and changing. This isn't always easy for others to do, especially initially.

When Loved Ones Invalidate You

One of the most frustrating and painful experiences that you've probably had many times as an emotionally sensitive adult, and that many of my students repeatedly report, is being invalidated by others when it comes to your intense emotional reactions and inability to tolerate distressing situations. And there will be times when this happens even as you continue to use and develop all the new skills you've been learning. Others may express through disapproval or downright dismissiveness that a situation that has caused you to become so derailed doesn't, from their perspective, truly warrant or justify the reactions you are exhibiting. You're looking for attention. You're looking for drama. You have to make a big huge deal out of everything. Eek! I just felt a knot in my stomach simply thinking about being spoken to in this way. It hurts!

When we receive this response, our nervous system becomes activated, and it makes our emotional pain exponentially worse. Telling emotionally sensitive people that they are wrong to feel something creates an inner sense of wretched turmoil and confusion that really can't adequately be described in words: *Because I am feeling this way. That's my reality. And you're trivializing it. It may not be a reaction that someone else would expect or find acceptable, but that's what's going on in my mind-body-spirit right now. This is my experience, whatever you might think!* When others invalidate you, they are not simply disagreeing with your point of view. It can be enough to make you feel invisible.

Deliberate invalidation is really just as cruel as telling a crying child to shut up because she has nothing to be sad about. (And unfortunately, this scenario has actually happened to many of us!) But the child *is* clearly sad. She learns that it's not okay to feel or, in the least, to show and share her vulnerable feelings. Of course, most people who invalidate us are not doing so to be intentionally cruel or abusive. They may even think they are being helpful by telling us to stop overreacting or to snap out of it, as if saying such things will somehow get us to come to our senses and undo our dysregulated state. There's a reason for everything, including others' reactions to our reaction. Some people are uncomfortable with the emotions that your emotions are bringing up in them and, therefore, as an act of self-defense and preservation, want to quickly shut the conversation down to avoid feeling or appearing vulnerable. They are essentially protecting themselves. But, whatever the reason and whether they intend to or not, invalidators are communicating through words and body language what we receive and interpret as *There is no merit to what you are feeling. Your point of view, thoughts, or emotions aren't legitimate and don't matter.* Ouch.

A Secret Recipe for Validation

The truth is that the person with BPD traits is, on a biological level, experiencing a disruption in clear thinking due to overactivity in different areas of her brain, including the amygdala, which activates the fear or fight-or-flight response, potentially causing her to become convinced that her thoughts and behaviors are justified (can be substantiated) by her intense emotions even when they are sometimes not (Aguirre and Galen 2013).

The person with BPD may not know how to convey what she needs in that desperate moment of emotional pain. But there is a secret recipe to help quell the incredible anxiety that a person with BPD feels when experiencing intense emotions. Although it may seem just too simple to be true, I have been both on the receiving and on the giving end of this recipe and, nine times out of ten, have experienced it as highly effective.

So, here it is. To be truly validating, you must genuinely and without judgment convey to the suffering person that you understand that she is feeling deeply and having the reaction she's having. That's it. Loved ones don't need to agree that the emotionally sensitive person's reaction is in proportion to or justified by the upsetting event. By giving validation, they are not compromising their integrity or lying or patronizing the suffering person. They are acknowledging that what's happening is her reality and that it's very real to her. You might consider sharing this tip with loved ones. It could make a real difference!

If you do, they are probably going to ask you to explain further or to give a good example of a validating statement, so here is one you can use: "I get that you're feeling really distraught about having forgotten to pick up the baking soda. Do you want to talk about it?" If their intention is to help you calm down and feel heard, let loved ones know that saying this is going to be far more effective than saying, "Really? Crying over baking soda? Get over it." And, again, it's not about other people pretending to agree with you or even believing that it is socially acceptable or the norm to cry uncontrollably on the kitchen floor because you forgot the baking soda. It's just about them acknowledging that they get that this *is* your experience in the moment and you are indeed experiencing that level of upset. It's real for you. They are acknowledging your experience of reality whether that reality makes sense to them or not. Most people don't know that this pretty simple act of validation can be incredibly soothing and comforting during our moments of suffering. To be heard. To be understood. To know that someone is aware of the level of intensity we are experiencing in that moment, whether it makes sense to us, to that person, or to anyone else.

So, to move forward with having healthier relationships with others as we're working on our issues with BPD and emotional sensitivity, we have to be willing to coach them on how to be more effective with us, and we need to continue to do healing work within. For many of us, this invalidation issue runs deep. In fact, we're often keenly aware that our past experiences of invalidation throughout childhood, adolescence, and even into adulthood impact how we perceive and navigate relationships today. Because of this, once you've become adept at managing day-to-day issues skillfully and have worked through your more imminent, present-day concerns, you may want to begin to move more deeply into the work of exploring the issues from your past that affect your ability to cope in the present. This next section will briefly touch upon the importance of healing old wounds so that we can have the relationships that we want today. But before going there, it's important to acknowledge that not everyone who has BPD or emotional sensitivity came from a dysfunctional home, though a great many of us have.

Healing Old Wounds

It is well known that one of the circumstances thought to cause a young child to develop borderline personality disorder is an invalidating home environment during the critical years of early childhood development. This can happen in many ways, including rejecting a child's attempt to express herself, shaming, punishing, or ignoring the child and thus causing her to suppress her natural emotional reactions, and telling the child that she is wrong for feeling a certain way. Of course, these types of responses are more of a reflection of the adult's inability to handle being present with and supportive of the child's emotional response, but that doesn't help the little girl who doesn't understand why mommy or daddy isn't coming to hug or otherwise comfort or soothe her when she wants or needs this.

For those of us who were told we were crybabies, weak, or wimps for allowing our emotions to show or for showing signs of being particularly sensitive, it can feel as if a wound is being ripped open and salt poured into it when, decades later as an adult, another adult tells us we are overreacting or being ridiculous when we are genuinely experiencing despair. The original emotional response increases tenfold, and after this further dysregulation, it can take a long time—often several hours or a day—for us to come back down to baseline.

The willingness of loved ones to learn about and practice validation is very often an essential ingredient in our recovery and well-being. However, we must accept the reality that they may not be receptive to understanding or participating skillfully in this process. When the other person is unwilling to even try, it may be time to start setting limits and reevaluating the relationship. In the meantime, you can practice validating yourself with compassion and nonjudgment in those moments when you are reacting intensely to distressing situations. Even saying things to yourself such as *I'm feeling really intensely in this moment, and that's understandable* or *I'm emotionally dysregulated* can help tremendously with deescalating the emotional intensity.

Dealing with Identity Issues

Self-validation can be a great solution when we need validation and aren't getting it from the outside. However, you may face another major challenge that many people with borderline personality disorder face when it comes to having healthy relationships: *identity disturbance.* If you suffer from this issue, you don't know who you are apart from other people. When this is the case, the question that then arises is *Who am I actually validating?*

For most people who do not have BPD, values, morals, or beliefs cannot easily be shaken or redirected at the drop of a hat, but for many of us, they often can. Not having you own set of values feeds into identity disturbance, because there is no anchor. We are adrift, being carried off and dramatically influenced by every new interaction, every new relationship, every new setting. Sure, you might have little inklings here and there about things you like and don't like, but your sense of self (who you are, what you believe in, your values, preferences, wishes, goals) can radically shift, often suddenly, depending on whose company you are keeping in a given moment.

You feel like a chameleon, a shape-shifter conforming to best fit into various social situations, to please others, and to be loved and accepted. Not knowing who you are or what you want leads to a sense of deep emptiness. It leads to a fear of being alone, because if you don't know who you are and you cling to others for a sense of self, it's quite unbearable to be alone. There's no one to look to for guidance on who to be. No cues. No one to mimic. No one to please. When you're not around other people, you may feel as if you don't really exist.

This experience of nonreality is sometimes called *depersonalization* in clinical circles, and it essentially means to feel disconnected. Aguirre and Galen (2015) note that depersonalization "happens when your emotions are so powerful that you disconnect from experiencing them" (92), and it can happen in those alone moments when you suffer from identity disturbance. This state can sometimes create urges to self-harm, during which you briefly feel pain, or bleed, to reassure yourself that you're really there. We know that such behaviors do not serve us and that we want to live our lives more skillfully in these dark moments.

I know about this phenomenon all too well. Identity disturbance is the symptom that led to my diagnosis of BPD. I told my psychiatrist that if all the people I knew were to gather in one room with me at the same time, I might explode. That's because I behaved so differently from one person to the next. I wouldn't know who or how to be. I'd be mortified. The thought was terrifying!

While I knew that I had this shape-shifting nature, most of the time it actually didn't present itself as an obvious problem. It seemed, instead, to help me fit in at different workplaces and in certain social groups, and it allowed me to present myself as the perfect partner to partners who were as different as night and day. It was how I survived and navigated the world, taking cues from those around me as to how I should behave, think, and feel. This all worked fine and dandy until I began to feel really unsettled with this lack of a sense of *me*. I began questioning how others could stand firm in beliefs, values, and preferences and not be swayed by others, no matter how convincing. I wondered how they could trust that standing their ground and being their own person wouldn't leave them cold and lonely and rejected. How they could trust that people would actually like them, even love them, not leave them. I wanted that, too.

Whenever I would occasionally experience glimpses of this desire, it felt like an indulgence in fantasy and not something I could realistically attain. Other people? Yes. For me? No. Otherwise I would have that by now, right? I'd ultimately quickly dismiss the desire and suppress it, because I had absolutely no idea that it is, in fact, possible to establish your own identity in adulthood, even after so many years of taking on the personalities of others. I thought I was stuck that way. I thought it was my destiny to be the female version of that character in *Catch Me If You Can*. The character, played by Leonardo DiCaprio, is an imposter who manipulates people for his own personal gain, pretending to be a different person to different people. But with

BPD, we're not pretending. We're not facetiously plotting our deception or maliciously manipulating.

For those who suffer from this symptom, it's part of the illness … but boy, did that character still somehow resonate, though my intentions have never been to purposely deceive or mislead. Even though it's not our intention, in response to experiencing identity disturbance issues, we may engage in behaviors that are perceived as manipulative. We're not being authentic. We don't know how. Sometimes we feel like crap because of this, but we don't know exactly why we're behaving this way or have any hope that we might be able to change. I could hardly contain myself when my psychiatrist told me that she thought DBT could help even with this. I could have my own personality! I could find out who I was. Finally!

If you are encouraged by this news like I was, you may also be afraid of what you might find as you set out to discover who you really are. I certainly wasn't sure that I'd like the real me, but it was a chance I was willing to take, reasoning that I could then work on those things that I didn't like. I certainly have been doing this, and so can you. For me, it has taken not only a lot of DBT practice but also a willingness to engage in intensive work in therapy, and the work has focused quite a bit on learning to reprogram some of the messages I received growing up that fed into my habit of people-pleasing and that fueled the cycles of my shifting personality. I had to challenge thoughts that I was inadequate, weak, and less than others and that I only deserved so much and would have to settle in most areas of my life.

A Wake-Up Call

As you read on, perhaps you'll relate and have some aha moments of your own, as the situation I'm about to share is unfortunately all too common. As a young girl, I repeatedly witnessed the adult women in my life changing their behaviors and preferences based on their partners at a given time—styles of music, clothing, whether or not they used drugs or drank, even whether or not they liked children, including their own—and these childhood and adolescent experiences had a major impact on me. I thought it was normal until I didn't anymore. In my thirties, I began to wake up to the fact that these women, now much older, were stuck in the same patterns, after all these years, still conforming and transforming and shape-shifting to please their partners. And it made me so sad. I realized I actually didn't really know who they were. Would I ever? They didn't even seem to know who they were.

I realized that I just couldn't allow myself to one day become like them. Even in the midst of my dysfunctional and maladaptive ways, and even though I threatened to kill myself over the years more times than I'd care to count, I still, deep down inside, loved life. I just didn't like the pain, and as an easily emotionally dysregulated person, I didn't know how to manage it. Yet, some inner, wiser part of me knew it would really be a shame to go on in patterns of denying my true self, whoever she might be.

Can you relate? Does this feel like a wake-up call? I know that I certainly needed one, and I got it. It came about ten years before it would make sense and I would actually begin to change my life, but it happened nonetheless. It came in the form of a quote sternly uttered by a coworker. I was in my mid-twenties and behaving like a total brat, completely sabotaging yet another job. My coworker said, "To thine own self be true." At the time, I rolled my eyes and dismissed him as some snooty-tooty, holier-than-thou jerk. And to be honest, I didn't know exactly what the words meant. It didn't land then, but that quote haunted me into my thirties as identity disturbance issues were becoming more troubling: *To thine own self be true.* Ah yes, some Shakespearean wisdom.

Well, you obviously can't be true to yourself when you don't know who you are, and that's where I was stuck back then and continued to be stuck until very recently in my life. I have decades of experience of not really knowing who I was. This showed up in almost every aspect of life, from seemingly innocuous things like always agreeing to go to the restaurant or movie that others suggested to weightier issues such as my religious beliefs and sexual orientation. Is any of this resonating with you? Do you ever find yourself doing this? I inevitably ended up taking on the mannerisms, opinions, and wishes of others, and I didn't have a self to whom I could be true. If a little voice inside whispered a preference of my own, I would usually, pretty much instantly and out of habit, squash it. Instead, I would go with the preferences of the person I was with in that moment.

This problem is more prevalent than you might think. There are examples of BPD traits throughout pop culture. There's actually a great example in the movie *Runaway Bride* with Julia Roberts. In it, a friend at a diner points out to Julia's character that she inevitably orders up her eggs the same way as whoever she is dating at the time does. If her new boyfriend orders his scrambled, she does too. New guy likes hard-boiled? That's her new favorite. Order up. She doesn't know what kind of eggs she prefers, and this illustrates all the other eggs in her life, so to speak. All the other areas where she takes on the preferences of the man in her life at the cost of her knowing and honoring who she is apart from him. Because the movie is a lighthearted Hollywood romantic comedy, it doesn't actually dig deeply into this implication, but the diner scene does provide us with an illustration of how identity disturbance can work in BPD.

For many of us, of course, the manifestations of identity disturbance are much more serious. Things that most people take for granted as being integral to who they are, such as religious beliefs, sexual orientation, political affiliation, and fundamental values, can all shift at a moment's notice, and the emotional and relationship consequences can be a heck of a lot heftier than adapting food choices to match someone else's. So how do we even begin to change this? To be truly successful in relationships, and in life, we need to know who we really are, and this is true whether or not we have identity disturbance, emotional sensitivity, or even BPD.

Discovering the Real You

To feel stable when you find yourself alone and to bring yourself into relationships whole, you must be willing to do the work to discover and befriend who you really are at the core. The goal is that eventually you'll start to feel comfortable and secure both when you are around others and when you're by yourself. There may be a part of you that thinks that spending time alone is absolutely impossible and not something you could ever tolerate. If so, please know that I have been there, have had the same thoughts, and yet have managed to emerge on the other side in victory. You can, too. Like me, you may actually grow to enjoy some alone time, something I never would have imagined possible. Please don't be discouraged!

So, how do you get there? In DBT, a major way to begin to explore who you really are, consistently and across situations and relationships, is to take a look at what you value. Identifying and honoring your values is part of the road map to self-discovery. At first, doing this may be difficult because you've grown accustomed to answering questions like "What do you think?" or "Which would you like?" on auto-response, based on cues from your environment and what you think will please the person asking the question. You must now ask yourself whether your responses are truly based on what you believe and want or whether you're coming up with answers that you think other people will want to hear, because you want to please them. It's going to take some hard work and practice, but it will truly be worth the effort.

Once you decide to behave in ways that are in alignment with your own personal values, you'll be well on your way to being you, no matter whose company you're keeping. When you find yourself in conversations or relationships with others who do not share your values, you'll then be able to choose to either act in a way that is skillful and in alignment with what matters most to you or go with the old unhealthy way of surrendering your own values and losing yourself. The more you practice, the stronger and more skillful you'll get. And even if you don't particularly struggle with identity disturbance but find that you are often passive and go along with other people's desires, only to bottle it all up and become resentful or angry, then identifying and committing to living your values can be helpful for you, too.

As you're practicing, you may find that you're looking for more resources to go deeper into this exciting process of self-exploration. I highly recommend a book titled *The Desire Map: A Guide to Creating Goals with Soul,* by Danielle LaPorte (2014). In it, the author often refers to her own emotional sensitivity as well as to techniques she has used to help identify and honor who she truly is at the core. She is not a psychiatric professional but rather an emotionally sensitive peer who has found her way and whose work is resonating with millions of people around the globe. She is one of those authentic voices who has figured out how to triumph over the challenges that emotional sensitivity can bring, so she is thriving, and not just surviving, as an emotionally sensitive person—something we all certainly aspire to achieve.

LaPorte proposes a revolutionary new way of setting goals that can really get us thinking about who we are and what we want out of life. She gets us to challenge the motivations behind those things we've been striving for up until now, challenging us to ask ourselves whether they are things we truly want or are what others have wanted for us or have told us that we should be pursuing. Her suggestion is to set goals with our "core desired feelings" in mind. This process can give us quite a bit of insight into our values and who we really are.

Choosing Your Values

Values make up a big part of who you are as a unique individual, and it's important to figure out what yours really are. As you work through this exercise, please simultaneously practice compassion for yourself. By now, you may have spent years taking on the values of others and adhering to and creating allegiances to philosophies and ways of being that didn't really feel right to you. Time and time again, you've known something has been off when you've seen how quickly you can shift these allegiances. There has been something deeply disconcerting about this, yet you couldn't pinpoint what it was or how to change it. You switched your perspectives so often that your seemingly inexplicable erratic behaviors actually do have at least one root cause: you haven't had a set of values to call your own. This is about to begin to change.

Once you identify your values, you can begin to align your actions with these values. For example, is honesty one of your values? That's a pretty common one. Is it very important to you that you are honest with others and that others are honest with you? What if you know that you value honesty, but you admit that you sometimes have a particularly difficult time being honest with your significant other? This then presents a good opportunity to work toward acting in greater alignment with your values. Perhaps you're afraid to tell your significant other the full scope of certain situations because you are afraid that you might be judged or, worse, left. But it nags at you, for you truly do want to be honest and trustworthy. This is an area for practice. This is an opportunity to honor who you really are: someone who values honesty and wants to be an honest person. As you begin to honor this part of yourself, by choosing to be honest even when it's inconvenient, it makes you vulnerable, or it's a bit of a risk, you become more confident in knowing who you are: *I am an honest person*. No matter who is in your space or what circumstance comes up, this is something you know to be true about yourself and can use to make decisions that will support your long- and short-term goals. It's part of your identity.

Real-World Activity:
Identifying Your Values

Look deep within and see if you can identify the values that you are committed to in your life or would like to be committed to. In your notebook, begin to explore and write about some of these values. What values are most important to you? Some examples of values are honesty, dependability, courage, humility, confidence, fairness, and assertiveness. If the words aren't coming to you right away, do a Google search for "lists of values," and you'll find a number of resources to work with for this assignment. As a start, jot down up to twenty values that you aspire to hold dear and practice.

Answer as honestly as you possibly can. Be as brave as you can. Check in with your body, mind, and spirit. Close your eyes and try to get in touch with what really feels right to you before you put down an answer. Perhaps for the first time, listen to that quiet voice that wishes to express an opinion or preference. Listen to your desire to be you. Your own self. Imagine that the people who will be in the room when you reveal these parts of yourself will love and accept you and not reject or judge you.

Do your very best to identify your values, because they are going to be essential markers and guideposts along the road to discovering and embracing your identity and becoming the person you truly want to be. Values are a bit like moral compasses. Once we know what our values are, we can then begin to make decisions that are in alignment with them, allowing us to feel like we are in integrity, because we are being true to ourselves and presenting this consistent self to all the people in our lives.

For a while, you may want to keep this list of your personal values handy and visible so that throughout the day you can remember what your values are. You can keep a copy on your phone, a printed list somewhere you'll see it (if you live alone, perhaps on the bathroom mirror), and maybe a copy in your glove compartment. As you encounter situations that are emotionally upsetting and you're faced with the choice of your next move, having this list of values handy will help.

In emotionally charged situations where your values will be challenged, it's important to remember what your values really are. I used to have a real issue with flirting with other men when I was already in a monogamous relationship. My boyfriend would call me out on it, noting that I did it even in his presence. While I was having a hard time being in integrity with the flirting issue (which hurt my boyfriend's feelings and eroded trust), I really wanted to be in integrity and honor my intention to cultivate the value of honesty, so I made a commitment to my boyfriend that I'd be more aware of this and work on stopping the flirting.

Sometimes he would ask me how my day was and ask how things were going with my goal. I had a difficult time refraining from flirting, and it broke my heart to be honest with him about my behavior, even though I had promised to do so. A few times I lied and said it was going well and that I wasn't flirting, because I didn't want to hurt him (and I value kindness), but then I would feel such unrest inside and guilt and shame for my dishonesty that I would confess. Although I felt embarrassed at the time, it was important to me that I be truthful with him. So I began choosing to prioritize honesty over kindness in those vulnerable moments, which was a difficult decision to make. Rather than lying to make my boyfriend happy, I was being true to myself and my values and honoring him through being honest. I was fortunate in that the consequences of my honesty were positive. It upset him temporarily when he heard the truth, but over time my boyfriend began to trust me more, and we grew closer. I also reduced and eventually stopped the flirting.

Think about some of the values you identified. How would you likely feel during and after a challenging situation if you disregarded your values? What are the potential consequences of doing so? Behaving skillfully and making interpersonal choices based on your values can help reduce emotional suffering for both you and others involved, creating more trust and more promising outcomes in relationships.

Paying Attention to How You Want to Feel

Keeping in mind how we want to feel not only clues us in more to who we really are but also creates yet another prompt for us to ask ourselves whether certain choices will likely elicit the outcomes we want or move us further away from them. For example, say the neighbor's dog keeps pooping on your doorstep. You open your door right now and find it's happened yet again. You're livid. You haven't said anything yet about the two other times it's happened and instead have resentfully cleaned it up and then passive-aggressively put it on the neighbor's doorstep.

Since the last time it happened, you've begun working on choosing behaviors that help you feel self-respect and that honor your newly identified values of behaving kindly and practicing self-compassion. When you see the poop again, your first urge is to march over there, shout at the neighbor to keep his dog out of your yard, and fling the poop at him like some of our primate relatives may be inclined to do in such a moment. But you're at a higher level of consciousness. You're changing. You're setting intentions and making new choices so that you can have new outcomes.

You might find yourself in a quandary. Will telling him off give you satisfaction in the moment and give you something to instantly do with all of that anger and adrenaline? Yeah. Probably. But ... will your shouting at your neighbor help you feel self-respect and tie into your value of kindness? Nope. Will not saying anything, passively allowing his offensive behavior to continue, and being passive-aggressive help you feel self-respect and tie into your value of self-compassion? Nope. If you're still not clear on how to respond, think not only about the sense of satisfaction you may feel in the moment that you unleash your rage on him but also about how you will likely feel afterward. Do you want to deal with the aftermath of shame and embarrassment?

I know firsthand that it's not easy work to deliberately slow things down and really think them through like this when you're that angry, but it will be much easier to do if you can get yourself calm before responding. Remember, the goal is to respond rather than react. I've literally gone into the bathroom and splashed my face with cold water to create a distraction and calm down before saying something in such a moment of emotional intensity. Once the emotion comes down a bit, you can think more rationally and reasonably. You can then work on figuring out the middle ground and proceed in a way that honors your new goals, how you want to feel, and the person you want to be.

Figuring Out Who You Are

Of course, figuring out who you are is far more complex than just identifying and adhering to your values, yet this is an excellent and powerful starting point that has set so many of us on this journey. Continuing to apply the other skills you've learned can further help. Mindfully sitting honestly with what you are feeling and thinking can assist you in better accepting who you really are and what's happening for you in a given moment, rather than pushing away reality or suppressing what you feel and the various things that make you who you are. Using skills to help tolerate distress can assist you in not making impulsive decisions that will take you out of feeling in integrity, and using skills to regulate emotions will help you take better care of yourself so that you have the emotional resiliency to do all of this work. All of these things help us develop a sense of authenticity and allow us to begin to recognize a sense of identity—our true self—apart from other people.

Identity disturbance—this feeling of being like a shape-shifting chameleon who doesn't know who she is—was the main BPD criteria that had me in emotional shambles. I couldn't imagine a day when I could really stay true to myself when I had spent my whole life mimicking others. Yet I have come not only to know who I am and feel comfortable in my own skin but also to honestly say that I love the person I know myself to be. I'm not perfect, and I still have work to do when it comes to consistently sticking to my values, but overall I am finally someone who, more often than not, is able to be herself across various situations and relationships. Before DBT, I never believed this could be possible, so if you also suffer from this particular issue, I have hope for you, too.

Black-and-White and Red Flags All Over

Have you ever really adored someone? Maybe put him on a pedestal, seeing him in an idealized way, as if he could do no wrong and were absolutely perfect? Until he did something that upset or disappointed you, and then suddenly, you couldn't stand him ... and (wham!) you pushed him off of that pedestal? He went from hero to zero in your opinion in two seconds flat? Whereas in one moment he was only good, in the next moment he was suddenly only bad and you wanted nothing more to do with him. I've been there, too, and as I'm sure you know, this behavior is no good for maintaining healthy relationships.

To reduce this behavior, so as not to damage our important relationships, we need to understand what's driving it. Sometimes our perception gets clouded, and we mistakenly see people and things in all-or-nothing, black-and-white terms and have difficulty seeing the shades of gray, or the middle ground. This can be a problem especially when we're feeling stressed. In other words, we might not notice important pieces of information and choices that are available to us in the moment, because we're thinking in extremes.

So where does the truth lie? Usually somewhere in the middle of those two extremes. Sometimes good people make mistakes or disappoint us, but they still remain good people in spite of this. They're imperfect, just like us. Practicing mindfulness by bringing our attention to when we are stuck in a faulty thinking pattern and giving ourselves the opportunity to challenge it can help foster our recovery in this area. The more we practice, the more aware we become. The awesome thing is that simply committing to being mindfully aware of these instances can help diminish their occurrence.

Real-World Activity:
Noticing Black-and-White Thinking

Create a section in your notebook specifically for noting those moments when you realize you've been stuck in black-and-white thinking. Write down some recent examples of when this kind of thinking has gotten in your way. In retrospect, what cues or red flags could you identify from your experience that might help you notice you're in this thinking style the next time it happens?

As you're practicing noticing and challenging black-and-white thinking, you will want to watch out for certain red flag words in your thoughts and speech, such as "never" and "always," as in "You never listen to me" or "You're always putting your job first." Rarely is anything truly in the *never* or *always* categories. If you find yourself making definitive statements like this, make it a goal to bring yourself into middle-ground thinking. For example, you might turn "You never listen to me" into "You're often preoccupied with watching sports on TV, and it hurts my feelings when I need to speak to you and you're unwilling to mute the sound and look in my direction." This reworking of the statement acknowledges that the other person sometimes listens, since you used the word "often" not "always" to describe the behavior that bothers you. That's more realistic in most cases and is less apt to put someone on the defensive and start an argument. Better to steer clear of the extremes.

It's also important to remember that other people are having their own experiences, and their outward expressions (a sigh, facial expression, choice of words, or tone of voice) may not be reactions or responses to you. If you check the facts (more on this topic shortly), and it turns out that they actually are behaving in a way that is less than sensitive, it will help to remember that no one is perfect. People will make mistakes and come up short. This doesn't negate all of the good they have done or instantly switch them from being a good person to a bad person. (Side note: This doesn't mean that you need to tolerate being treated poorly. You can do your best to use the skills you've learned so far to assertively express your concerns without losing your self-respect or damaging the relationship.)

Likewise, if you make a mistake or fall short, this does not negate all of the hard work you've been doing or instantly switch you from a hardworking good person to a bad person or make you a failure. A mistake or a setback does not define you, just as these things do not define someone else.

Whenever you find yourself feeling trapped because there seem to be only two extreme options available to you, consider that you might be caught up in black-and-white thinking, and then try to come up with some other possible solutions and options. I am finally beginning to have more breakthroughs in this area, and I recently tweeted out this epiphany: "Just because I cannot see another possibility or solution in this moment doesn't mean it doesn't exist." Whether it's a relationship-based thought or any other thought where we are able to see only two starkly opposite, seemingly incompatible options or solutions, if we work hard, we can find those shades of gray and realize that we do, in fact, have more options.

Become a Fact Checker

As previously mentioned, it can sometimes be helpful to check the facts in fraught situations where the facts may not be as obvious as they first appear. For this, you may need to conjure up your favorite detective. Are you old enough to remember Columbo? Maybe Mulder or Scully are more your style? Sherlock? Think about how your chosen character typically goes about getting to the bottom of things. What methodology is used for finding the truth in situations?

Think about how the detective may be initially swayed by past experiences and judgments in figuring out what happened. While a first hunch may be correct, more often than not the cases have twists and turns that result in a different outcome or solution. Keeping this perspective in mind can help you more skillfully engage in your relationships with others, since this is how life generally works too. While we can learn from the past and use historical information to help us navigate new situations, we can't count on things always turning out the same way. There will always be different variables: different people, different circumstances. Heck, you've grown and evolved and are different from the person you were in previous relationships!

That being said, two things that have likely remained consistent for you are being emotionally sensitive and tending to suffer in connection with some (or many) BPD traits. Both of these factors can color our world—our perceptions, interpretations, thoughts, and beliefs—and therefore how we relate to other people in relationships. In addition, if we have been hurt in the past or have suffered trauma, our nervous systems can be activated by our reactions to things as seemingly slight as a facial expression, sigh, or tone of voice. We can become anxious or even terrified, believing that a roll of the eyes most definitely means that someone is going to leave us forever.

We might become furiously angry because our boyfriend breaks eye contact or rolls his eyes when asked if he's cheating, since the thought *He must be cheating* feels so strong in that moment, and we think it must be true (even if there is no evidence beyond said eye rolling to support this). Our interpretations and insecurities about what people mean by a look they've given us or the words they have chosen are intensified even more if we are feeling less resilient emotionally because of stress.

How do we avoid our old knee-jerk reactions? In the case of distorted thoughts around others' intentions, we can make real headway. Fact-checking challenges us to not believe our thoughts and interpretations at face value but to actually, like a detective, do some investigational work to determine if our thoughts are indeed accurate.

So many of us with BPD react to others based on our sometimes inaccurate interpretations. Say your loved one just got home from work. You're so glad to see him and you start telling him all about your day. While you're midsentence, he plops down in a chair in front of the computer, lets out a huge sigh, and then barely utters, "Uh, huh," as he stares at the monitor and reaches for the mouse. A sense of dread arises in the pit of your stomach. You feel crushed. Your thoughts have jumped to *He's no longer interested in me. He doesn't care. This relationship is over. He's going to leave! He's already made up his mind!*

Your eyes well up with tears, and you storm off, slamming the door behind you.

"What?" your loved one calls out as he jumps up from his chair and follows you into the next room. "What is it? What happened? What did I do?" Now you've got his attention.

"Don't play dumb," you snap back. "You wanna leave? Go. Just take your stuff and get the *#&$ out of here before I call the cops and have them take you away."

Your loved one stands there frozen, stunned, and confused and really concerned about your mental well-being.

Notice in this scenario that you had no actual, factual evidence that your loved one had plans or a desire to leave. You heard him sigh and seem disinterested, and you leapt to a conclusion. You then began to *believe* and then *behave* in accordance with this conclusion, not taking the time to check whether your thoughts were accurate. Your loved one's reaction was one of complete bewilderment and fear. Familiar scene? It was for me, many, many times in the past!

So, how can we be skillful if we want to work on not mindlessly believing and reacting to our emotionally charged thoughts, knowing that they are sometimes not accurate representations of reality? We can begin by asking ourselves in the moment how accurate a thought most likely is, given context clues, and by coming out and asking questions. This approach takes a willingness to experience a certain level of vulnerability. Some of our thoughts may come off as "out there" to someone who doesn't have our type of history. Our thoughts may very well be off the mark or may sound flat-out paranoid to others. ("Uhm, are you leaving me and breaking up this marriage, and that's why you sighed and looked the other way?") But before fact-checking by asking questions of someone we trust, we can disclose that we realize we may be off the mark and that we are working on being more skillful about not jumping to conclusions.

Call upon your inner detective, and ask, for example, "I know this may sound out there, but I'm working on fact-checking instead of believing and mindlessly reacting to everything I think. I'm just going to ask, did you just sigh because you don't love me anymore and are planning on leaving me?" If he responds judgmentally with something along the lines of "How in the world could you think that? Are you out of your mind?" even after you made your earlier disclaimer, it could be helpful to show a sense of humor. You could say, "I'm not sure. That's why I'm taking the time to check my thoughts, thank you." I sometimes remind people that I have a trauma history that may inaccurately color my perception of reality and that I'm working on that, too. People are sometimes more compassionate and understanding when they have a sense of the *why*, a reasonable explanation behind what they consider to be odd behavior.

The other person will usually answer that our extreme, emotionally charged thought is not accurate or at least not entirely accurate. For example, your loved one may confess that he was uninterested in talking right when he came home from work, because he'd had a hard day and needed to rest and recharge before having the mental bandwidth to have an engaged discussion. "No, I don't want to leave you, and I still love you. I just need some time to decompress, relax, do my thing, surf the Net for an hour or so. Then I can be myself and talk about whatever you'd like." In this scenario, it's very unlikely that you're now crying, storming off, or in hysterics worrying that he's about to pack his bags. All because you took the time to fact-check.

No Leads on the Case?

What if your thought is that you are going to lose your job, and your fear is so high that you think it must be true? You think this is true because your boss has been moody lately, and you're beginning to behave and react as if you've already been fired. You can't really check the facts by asking your boss if your thought is true. So what can you do in this situation? In such situations, your detective work could include talking to other people you trust, including your therapist if you are seeing someone. Ask for a reality check during which you will share your thoughts uncensored. You also can do a reality check on your own, in which you rate the likelihood of your thought having merit and actually happening. Here's how to do it.

Real-World Activity:
Reality Check

The next time you are afraid something bad will happen and want to examine the evidence for it happening, take out your notebook and write down what you fear will happen. Then write out why you think it's going to happen, and document evidence for and against these thoughts being true. Then, on a scale of 0 to 100 percent possibility, rate the likelihood that what you fear happening will come true. Here's an example.

Thought: *I'm afraid I'm going to get fired. My boss has been moody lately, and I can just feel it in my bones. I'm so scared. I may as well just get my stuff and leave. I may just give him a piece of my mind on my way out, too.*

Examining the evidence: *Well, I'm terribly afraid and anxious, so part of me thinks that this is a sign or an indication that it must be true … that I'm just doomed. But actually my boss has been moody with everyone. I recently had a good review, and I've been here for years. I have a set of skills that not many people have, so it's unlikely they would let me go. All things considered, I think it's my fear talking more than anything. The actual likelihood that I am truly going to get fired at this point is probably pretty low, maybe 5 percent if my boss were someone who acted on pure emotion due to his moodiness. I probably don't have anything to worry about.*

This exercise can help you look with more objectivity at upsetting and oftentimes inaccurate thoughts.

Sometimes I have felt silly for even getting so intensely upset about a thought that, once spoken, written down, and rated on a scale, seemed so unlikely. I wondered how I could have been so affected by it. If this happens to you, it's important not to judge yourself. Instead, you can acknowledge that you took the time to skillfully approach the issue rather than go the old route of simply believing a thought and dealing with the consequences of acting on it. This takes work, and no one can do it for you. It really is an accomplishment when you choose to respond skillfully.

Relationships Are Complicated

You know how complicated relationships can be and especially with the added complications and challenges brought on by BPD and emotional sensitivity. Now you have some new skills to experiment with and to use to empower yourself to be more skillful in the relationships most important to you. This is by no means a comprehensive set of tools, but it is a really good start when combined with all of the other skills you've learned in this book.

My advice is to take it one moment at a time. Check in with yourself to see how you're feeling, and always keep in mind your ultimate goals in your relationships. When you feel the urge to act in a way that is unlikely to be effective in moving toward your goals, take the time to seriously consider the potential consequences and how a moment of satisfaction or relief from self-destructive behaviors just isn't worth the suffering that comes with these types of choices in the long run. You've done a lot of work throughout these chapters. I hope you are very proud of yourself. Now let's put this all together.

Chapter 5

Putting It All Together

We've been on this journey together for a while now, so I want to update you on a little moment of success that I recently experienced. I hope it will encourage you as we wrap things up.

Remember that guy from work who said, "To thine own self be true"? The last time I'd seen him was in my twenties, before I had discovered DBT and started on this healing path. Then recently I bumped into him again. I had stopped at a grocery store that was several hours away from the town where we both lived and worked years ago. It was such an unlikely meeting that I imagine that the Universe must have deliberately set up the opportunity. It felt like a gift.

And no, I didn't run and hide in a crowded aisle to avoid him and feel shame for my past or for the old me who shared an office with him years ago. Instead, I felt a sense of peace. There he was with his baby and his wife. When he saw me, the look on his face was one of surprise. I smiled at him, and then the words just flowed. I took the opportunity to thank him for saying what he did that day and told him that I finally understood the quote.

Kind of nice. Thank you again, and thank you, William Shakespeare: "To thine own self be true."

To you and all of the emotionally sensitive souls, those with BPD and those with BPD traits, working so hard to overcome the challenges in this life, may you know that life has these types of moments in store for you, too. May you know that there is hope. May you find and stay true to the real you and live the life you were meant to live. May you continue to be encouraged to practice and live the skills you've learned in this book, to learn even more skills, and to stick with it.

This book may be the first of many steps or one in a series in your ongoing path of progress toward healing. Yours is a unique journey. Keep in mind that no two recoveries will ever look the same. Remember that you are going to get out of it what you put in, and there are going to be times when you will just want to give up. Don't.

We each have a purpose to fulfill. A meaningful role to play on this earth. You are a vital piece in the big puzzle of humanity. You matter. Your story, your heart, your love, your experiences. All of you.

Yes, there will be difficult times, and yes, life can be painful. You've now learned that the old adage is true: pain is inevitable, but suffering is optional. Where once you may have had very little insight or the drive or encouragement or information that you needed to make skillful choices, you're now in a different place. You have some tools that you can begin using as you further pursue your DBT studies and get the support you need to enter into or maintain recovery.

You have a number of skills to call upon to help you be more mindful in your world, to more fully appreciate each moment and more fully experience your life. You have skills to help you slow down and engage in healthy behaviors that won't make matters worse when you're in a crisis or stressing and there isn't an immediate solution to your problem. You've learned some ways to take care of yourself and learned how doing so can impact and support how you feel emotionally. And you've learned some skills to support your efforts when it comes to creating, maintaining, and repairing important relationships. You're not the same person who picked up this book and started reading it. You're growing and evolving. Yes, you're already beginning to change!

It took willingness and perseverance to make it through these chapters and to take an honest personal inventory all along the way. It's difficult to really examine ourselves, especially when we are not pleased with what we see in the moment. It took courage to begin challenging your thoughts and choices and to consider your role in situations and relationships that were not working as well as you would have liked. And the journey continues. With continued willingness, you'll expand your understanding and practice of DBT skills and develop more skills. You'll have more resources to call upon to continue to improve your life and live the way you'd like.

Keep it up. Know that you are never alone. We are all on this journey together.

To thine own self be true. Stay skillful.

In kindness,

Debbie

Thank You

G.: Thank you for loving me through my darkest times and always encouraging me to believe in myself. You are my biggest cheerleader. You said I should do something with my writing. I have. Your friendship and support mean the world to me. We are Jerry and Elaine. Love you forever. Thank you.

SL: Thank you for being such a good friend and teaching me how to trust in my ability to be a good friend, too. Thank you for also teaching me how to be in and feel safe in my body and to listen to my Spirit. Love you.

KD: Thank you for being there for me like only you can. There are some things that only you understand. E e! Best friends forever, even if we fight (yeah!). I love you.

F&B aka "the boys": I love you! You are the most nonjudgmental healers.

RD: Thank you for doing your best and for your thoughtful ways. I love you.

Nana, Grandma, Daddy, and FC: I miss you. Thank you for the love you gave me.

AB, SB, and little GG: So glad you are all now in my life. Yay for technology!

MBG: Thank you for everything! You continue to make such a difference in my life.

VH: Thank you for your ongoing support throughout the years.

FK: Thank you for always encouraging and believing in the best of me.

SG: Our work together helped me have breakthroughs. Thank you.

Kiera Van Gelder: Thank you for your inspiration and encouragement.

Gillian Galen: Thank you for your clinical insights and your help and encouragement through the entire process of writing this book.

Jess, Caleb, Brady, and the entire New Harbinger team: Thank you for helping me become more of a critical thinker in my writing and a stronger writer overall.

Amanda Smith: Thank you for being a friend and an inspiration!

Thank you to the staff and other young adults I met in the group homes I was in as a teen in Massachusetts. The experiences I had with you changed my life for the better.

Thank you to the caring, amazing staff at the emergency and psychiatry departments of the many Northern California Kaiser Permanente facilities where I've received services.

Thank you to the talk radio show personalities at KGO 810 AM in San Francisco, especially Ronn Owens. Listening to you over the years has been a source of comfort and enlightenment and has helped me get through some difficult times. You've turned me into a talk radio junkie. Thank you for doing what you do.

Dr. Marsha Linehan: Thank you for listening to your calling, courageously and strongly working through and overcoming your own challenges, and for creating a modality that has saved my life and the lives of countless others. I am forever grateful.

Thank you, Oprah Winfrey and Iyanla Vanzant, for serving as the strong female role models I so desperately needed in my life. Because of your willingness to shine your lights, I along with so many others have been afforded the opportunity to learn so much from your teachings. I am forever grateful for all that you do for humanity.

Thank you to the Universe for supporting me through my metamorphosis and reminding me that I am made of the same stuff as the stars and that I matter.

Thank you to my blog readers and students. You inspire and encourage me every day.

Thank you.

References

Aguirre, B., and G. Galen. 2013. *Mindfulness for Borderline Personality Disorder: Relieve Your Suffering Using the Core Skill of Dialectical Behavior Therapy.* Oakland, CA: New Harbinger Publications.

———. 2015. *Coping with BPD: DBT and CBT Skills to Soothe the Symptoms of Borderline Personality Disorder.* Oakland, CA: New Harbinger Publications.

Bassett, L. 2006. *Attacking Anxiety and Depression Program, a Drug-Free, Self-Help Guide to Curing Anxiety, Depression and Stress.* Multimedia CD. Los Angeles: Midwest Center.

LaPorte, D. 2014. *The Desire Map: A Guide to Creating Goals with Soul.* Boulder, CO: Sounds True.

Linehan, M. M. 1993a. *Cognitive Behavioral Treatment of Borderline Personality Disorder.* New York: Guilford Press.

———. 1993b. *DBT Skills Training Manual.* New York: Guilford Press.

———. 2014a. *DBT Skills Training Handouts and Worksheets.* 2nd ed. New York: Guilford Press.

————. 2014b. *DBT Skills Training Manual.* 2nd ed. New York: Guilford Press.

McKay, M., J. C. Wood, and J. Brantley. 2007. *The Dialectical Behavior Therapy Skills Workbook: Practical DBT Exercises for Learning Mindfulness, Interpersonal Effectiveness, Emotion Regulation, and Distress Tolerance.* Oakland, CA: New Harbinger Publications.

Debbie Corso is a mental health blogging pioneer, courageously chronicling her journey while lighting a torch to provide hope to a severely emotionally wounded community. She has a BS from New York Institute of Technology in interdisciplinary studies in behavioral science, communications, and English, as well as a certificate in early childhood development. She is in recovery from borderline personality disorder (BPD). Through hard, consistent work with dialectical behavior therapy (DBT), she no longer meets the criteria to be considered "borderline." Her work as an intake coordinator and case manager at a non-profit organization, working closely with children at risk for abuse and neglect, was the catalyst that propelled her to document and share her powerful journey through her blog, and hopeful and encouraging books on overcoming the oppressive symptoms of BPD. She currently cofacilitates online, worldwide DBT psycho-educational courses at www.emotionallysensitive.com. She lives in the San Francisco Bay Area.

Foreword writer **Gillian Galen, PsyD**, is instructor of psychology at Harvard Medical School. She is program director and assistant director of training for McLean 3East Intensive Residential Program at the Harvard-affiliated McLean Hospital—a unique residential DBT program for young women exhibiting self-endangering behaviors and BPD traits. She specializes in adolescent psychotherapy, including DBT. She has a particular interest in using mindfulness and yoga in the treatment of BPD and other psychiatric illnesses. Galen has been a registered yoga instructor since 2008. She is coauthor of *Mindfulness for Borderline Personality Disorder*.

FROM OUR PUBLISHER—

As the publisher at New Harbinger and a clinical psychologist since 1978, I know that emotional problems are best helped with evidence-based therapies. These are the treatments derived from scientific research (randomized controlled trials) that show what works. Whether these treatments are delivered by trained clinicians or found in a self-help book, they are designed to provide you with proven strategies to overcome your problem.

Therapies that aren't evidence-based—whether offered by clinicians or in books—are much less likely to help. In fact, therapies that aren't guided by science may not help you at all. That's why this New Harbinger book is based on scientific evidence that the treatment can relieve emotional pain.

This is important: if this book isn't enough, and you need the help of a skilled therapist, use the following resources to find a clinician trained in the evidence-based protocols appropriate for your problem. And if you need more support—a community that understands what you're going through and can show you ways to cope—resources for that are provided below, as well.

Real help is available for the problems you have been struggling with. The skills you can learn from evidence-based therapies will change your life.

Matthew McKay, PhD
Publisher, New Harbinger Publications

If you need a therapist, the following organization can help you find a therapist trained in dialectical behavior therapy (DBT).

Behavioral Tech, LLC
please visit www.behavioraltech.org and click on *Find a DBT Therapist.*

For additional support for patients, family, and friends, contact the following:

BPD Central **Visit www.bpdcentral.org**

Treatment and Research Advancements Association for Personality Disorder (TARA)
Visit www.tara4bpd.org

National Alliance on Mental Illness (NAMI) **Please visit www.nami.org**

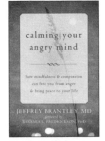
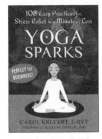
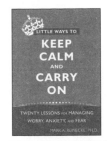
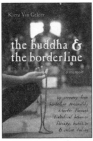
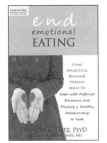
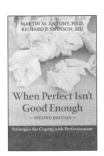 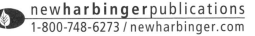